Kris Swanson
543-8228

Surviving Pregnancy Loss

Surviving *Pregnancy Loss*

ROCHELLE FRIEDMAN, M.D.
BONNIE GRADSTEIN, M.P.H.

LITTLE, BROWN AND COMPANY — BOSTON – TORONTO

First edition

The authors are grateful to the *American Journal of Nursing* for
permission to quote excerpts from an article by Carol Hard-
grove and Louise Warrick entitled "How Shall We Tell the
Children," which appeared in the *American Journal of Nursing* in
March, 1974. Copyright © 1974 by the *American Journal of
Nursing*.

LIBRARY OF CONGRESS CATALOGING IN PUBLICATION DATA
Friedman, Rochelle.
  Surviving pregnancy loss.
  Bibliography: p.
  Includes index.
  1. Miscarriage—Psychological aspects. 2. Still birth—Psychological as-
pects. 3. Pregnancy, Ectopic—Psychological aspects. 4. Loss (Psychol-
ogy) 5. Pregnancy—Psychological aspects. I. Gradstein, Bonnie. II.
Title.
    RG648.F74   155.9'37   82-7216
    ISBN 0-316-29349-0   AACR2

BP
Designed by Susan Windheim
Published simultaneously in Canada
by Little, Brown & Company (Canada) Limited

Printed in the United States of America

Foreword

Very few pregnant women anticipate an outcome to their pregnancy that is less than perfect. Vital statistics indicate, however, that this view may be too optimistic. Fifteen of every hundred pregnancies end in a spontaneous abortion (miscarriage), another one in eighty ends in the delivery of a dead infant, while still another one in a hundred is an ectopic pregnancy. All three of these complications deprive the woman of her expected child and evoke in her and her husband feelings of loss, grief, and anger.

Unfortunately, the physician's focus on the physical problems associated with the loss of the pregnancy can interfere with his or her ability to recognize and deal with the emotional needs of the couple. A physician's usual response to a miscarriage is to inform the woman that it is a common occurrence and is nature's way of eliminating potentially abnormal individuals. This explanation, while accurate, does not deal with the couple's perception that their baby has been lost and their emotional response to that perception. Ectopic pregnancy is still a cause of maternal deaths in this country because of internal hemorrhage. For that reason, it is with a sense of relief that a physician completes the successful surgical treatment of an ectopic pregnancy. Preserving the mother's life is the paramount concern. Surgery relieves the woman of the pain associated with the ectopic pregnancy, but then she must face not only the loss of her baby, but the realization that her chances for successful pregnancy in the future are decreased substantially. Often these concerns are not addressed by physicians because of their concentration on the surgery and the physical recovery that follows it.

When confronted by pregnancy loss, friends and relatives tend to fall back on clichés that do little to assuage the couple's grief. "It's all for the best," "The baby would have been abnormal...," "You'll be pregnant again soon and will have no problems" are poor substitutes for what the couple really needs — a chance to ventilate their grief. A major problem is that others do not perceive a miscarriage or ectopic pregnancy as loss of a child, whereas the couple experiences the loss often as strongly as they would the stillbirth of a full-term infant.

The response of health care professionals to the emotional needs of couples who have experienced a stillbirth has improved dramatically in the last decade. Many hospitals have specific individuals trained to help parents deal with their need to grieve and to ventilate their feelings. Follow-up sessions are provided even after the woman is discharged from the hospital, and couples are encouraged to join groups made up of individuals who have sustained similar pregnancy losses. Even with these aids couples still must rely primarily on their own psychological and emotional resources. This is especially true in today's society, where families are atomized and close relatives may be thousands of miles away.

On rare occasions a book is published that provides crucial information for both patients and their physicians. Norman Cousins's *Anatomy of an Illness* and Martha Lear's *Heartsounds* are two recent examples. *Surviving Pregnancy Loss* is another. For the individual who has suffered a pregnancy loss it shows that others have had similar experiences, similar grief, and similar emotional reactions. The book performs a vital service by bringing to the fore the realization that it is not just the wife who is traumatized. The husband too suffers and he is under the added burden of societal expectations that he will keep a stiff upper lip. This book contains not only descriptions of reactions to pregnancy loss, but also practical approaches to coping with the associated emotional problems. I cannot emphasize the last point too strongly. Couples need help, and *Surviving Pregnancy Loss* is uniquely suited to provide that help. For the physician, it will aid in understanding the emotional needs of individuals who have had a miscarriage, an ectopic pregnancy, or a stillbirth. For most physicians it will be a revelation to learn that couples can regard an ectopic pregnancy as the loss of a baby.

Let there be no mistake; the book is not a depressant. The stories told by the individuals who have lost a pregnancy are moving and evoke in the reader an admiration for the spirit of these individuals as they cope with their adversity. Moreover, the suggestions for coping provide a realistic plan for escaping the depression associated with the loss of a baby. Last, there is a wonderful chapter on adoption that demonstrates that there are alternatives even for those couples who choose not to risk the potential disappointment of another pregnancy.

Both Dr. Friedman, who is a psychiatrist, and Mrs. Gradstein, who has a master's degree in public health and is a counselor in the area of reproduction, have had extensive experience in working with couples who have experienced pregnancy loss. Their advice is sympathetic and, most important, it is practical. It also is clearly written and free of jargon.

Who should read this book? Everyone who has had a miscarriage, an ectopic pregnancy, or a stillbirth; anyone who has a friend or relative who has had a pregnancy loss; every physician; and, finally, anyone who wants to understand the stresses placed on the human spirit by loss of a baby, and the resiliency of individuals in coping with that misfortune.

ROBERT H. GLASS, M.D.
Professor
Obstetrics, Gynecology and Reproductive Sciences
University of California, San Francisco

Foreword

Nothing I had learned in thirty years of living prepared me for the loss of my first pregnancy. After several years of longing, I had finally conceived a child. My joy knew no bounds. Thirteen weeks later I lay bleeding in the hospital, a miscarriage "statistic." I was discharged home a day later, physically well, but not well at all. Life went on (yes, they tell me it did) but I was lost in a limbo of half-grief, in a place that knows death but has no rituals or rites for comforting. People said all the wrong things. They said it was nature's way, that the baby would not have been normal. They told me I would be pregnant again in no time. No one seemed to know what I felt. There were no books to read, to see if my reactions were normal. Women were all around me, but I had no way to locate those who could share this experience. My husband and I were locked in separate circles of grief, unable to communicate to each other. This was one of the loneliest times of my life.

It was to be my only pregnancy. I went on to build a family, not through birth, but by adoption. I also went on to start an organization for people suffering from infertility and pregnancy loss. RESOLVE is now in its ninth year and has grown to become a national consumer advocacy organization for infertile couples, with thirty-eight chapters around the country. In each chapter we offer counseling and support groups. We help couples who have experienced infertility and pregnancy loss to find each other, and to ease the pain with the caring concern of those who have been there.

The authors of this exceptional book have been there, through personal experience and their collective professional experience. I am pleased that many of the vivid anecdotal pieces that enrich the text came from members of RESOLVE who responded to a request put in our national newsletter. That request also brought these two authors together. I feel the pride of an honorary midwife that the collaborative effort was facilitated through my work at RESOLVE.

This book is largely about the feelings surrounding pregnancy loss. We see chronicled not just the initial and necessary feelings of guilt and anger and grief, but the ultimate feelings of acceptance, of courage to try again, and of victory over despair. A special section on the male partner reveals the unique and different patterns men may use in grieving for lost progeny and (sometimes) confronting a threat to the life of their partner.

I recommend this book for all couples who are facing, or who have faced, the experience of pregnancy loss. There is information here, and validation for their feelings. They are not alone; they can be comforted by the experience of others. I particularly recommend this book to all helping professionals who may come in contact with couples experiencing pregnancy loss. Since it is not possible for professionals to counsel about only what they have experienced in life, the next best thing is for them to walk a mile in our shoes. This book will provide all who read it with valuable insights into the experience of and recovery from pregnancy loss.

BARBARA ECK MENNING
Executive Director, RESOLVE

Preface

Every book has a story, and every story has a beginning. *Surviving Pregnancy Loss* is somewhat unusual in that it had two beginnings. Through our own very different experiences, each of us became aware of the need for a book that would help people who had been through the loss of a pregnancy understand what had happened, cope with the loss, and plan for the future.

Dr. Rochelle Friedman's interest in working with individuals who have experienced the loss of a pregnancy dates back to the early 1970s. Until that time neither the medical nor the psychological profession had paid a great deal of attention to the many emotional and physical health problems that primarily or exclusively affect women. However, by the early 1970s that situation was starting to change in response to pressure from the women's movement as well as to increasing interest within the professions in the normal life experiences of both women and men. In this climate of opinion, old notions about women were starting to break down and a generation of articulate, concerned women was beginning to educate society about what women's health needs really were.

In 1973, one such woman, a fifty-five-year-old teacher, sought counseling for a long-standing depression. In the course of talking about her life, she recounted in minute detail the events surrounding a miscarriage she had experienced some thirty years before. Her account raised important questions: why was it that a loss so profound that it was recalled moment by moment after years had gone by been virtually ignored in medical and psychiatric training? Why had a problem that affected so many people been overlooked?

A search of the medical and lay literature confirmed the suspicion that little attention had been paid to the subject of pregnancy loss. The medical literature held only a few articles on the subject, most of them in nursing journals. The psychiatric literature was even more disappointing: all that could be found were studies and observations purporting to demonstrate that pregnancy loss is related to a woman's conflicts, whether about her femininity or about her wish for a child. As for the lay literature, there was a profusion of books that dealt with the "healthy pregnancy," but only very few that included anything at all about the complications of pregnancy or about pregnancy loss. Similarly, a fairly extensive search turned up few resources: little in the way of support services and very few health professionals who saw the need to pay attention to anything other than the physical aspects of pregnancy loss.

The decision was made to find out more about what the individual who has lost a pregnancy experiences and how best to meet the needs of this population. In 1976 a postmiscarriage peer support group was organized at the Massachusetts Institute of Technology, with five women participating. The group was led jointly by Dr Friedman and Ms. Karen Cohen, then a health educator at M.I.T. The group was conceived of as being both therapeutic and educational. The goal of the educational component was to help women understand what had happened to them, so that they could achieve intellectual mastery over an event that they had initially experienced as overwhelming. The brief psychotherapy was designed to help the participants examine their experiences with pregnancy, to explore their feelings about the loss of their pregnancies, and to help them resolve their loss.

During the course of meeting together to share experiences, concerns, and support, it became clear that, although the exact circumstances of each woman's miscarriage were different from those of any other, there were many common aspects. Each of the participants had discovered that although family, friends, and medical helpers had all minimized her loss, there was a community of people who understood what they had been through. The women learned that they were not overreacting to a trivial loss, as they had been led to believe. On the contrary, they came to realize that they had been experiencing feelings of sadness and disappointment because they were mourning the loss of a specific irreplaceable and valued pregnancy.

As professionals, we learned that most women form an attach-

ment to the fetus far earlier in the pregnancy than we had previously thought; that the child who will never be is mourned; and
that the mourning process that follows the loss of a pregnancy,
even an early loss, resembles that experienced when a beloved person dies. We also learned that no group of experts exists to help
people through the crisis of losing a pregnancy, and, in fact, the
true experts are those people who have themselves experienced
such a loss. The decision to write a book by and for people who had
been through this trauma developed out of this background.

Surviving Pregnancy Loss is based on clinical work with many men
and women who have experienced infertility or suffered the loss of
a pregnancy. It is also based on information gathered through a
searching questionnaire that was completed by more than sixty
women who had experienced the loss of one or more pregnancies.
Participants were recruited through advertisements placed in the
national newsletter of RESOLVE, an organization serving the
needs of people with infertility problems, and in the national
newsletter of OURS, a support group for adoptive parents.

In addition to the many responses, which you will find throughout this book in the form of quotations, shared experiences, and
suggestions for coping, the ad yielded two completely unforeseen
benefits. First, a lengthy personal narrative describing her own
stillbirth was received from Charlene Arcidiacono. Reading about
Mrs. Arcidiacono's experience made it clear that the best way to
learn about what the loss of a pregnancy is really like is to hear
about it from someone who has been through it. Mrs. Arcidiacono's account can be found in the section on stillbirth, "One
Woman's Experience."

The "request for contact" notice in the RESOLVE newsletter
also yielded a telephone call from Bonnie Gradstein, a woman who
was deeply interested and involved in the area of pregnancy loss.
In addition to having lost two pregnancies herself, she was a professional counselor who often dealt with other women who were
coping with pregnancy loss. After many hours on the phone between Boston and San Francisco, it became clear to both of us that
we had to write this book together. Thus our collaboration began.

Mrs. Gradstein's belief that a book about what it was really like
to lose a pregnancy was long overdue, her vast experience in the

field of reproductive-health counseling, and her own experiences make her the natural person to collaborate on the kind of book that she wishes had been available to her when she needed it.

Mrs. Gradstein acquired a firsthand knowledge of how lonely, baffling, and agonizing the loss of a pregnancy could be when her first pregnancy ended in miscarriage and her second with the birth of a stillborn child. Although she was lucky in many respects, for her family and friends were loving and supportive, for the first time in her life she felt totally alone, empty, and out of control. She remembers walking around in a fog, sad and uncomprehending, wondering why she felt so bad, if she was crazy, and if her life was really falling apart. Although she managed to survive the experience, it was the hardest thing she had ever had to face. The struggle was a lonely one: there was nothing out there to help her — no books to read, no one to tell her she would make it.

As a result of these two losses, the focus of her career as a counselor changed significantly. Whereas in the past most of the women she had worked with had gone on to have healthy babies, now she was led to try to meet the needs of a different group, one for whom there was no existing support system: couples who had problems with having babies, some who had difficulty conceiving and others who were unable to carry a pregnancy to term.

Also, as a result of their own experience in adopting a child, Mrs. Gradstein and her husband, Marc, a practicing attorney, learned a great deal about private adoption. With the encouragement and support of the Department of Obstetrics, Gynecology and Reproductive Sciences at the University of California, San Francisco, for the past five years they have been educating people about private adoption, as well as guiding many through the private adoption process.

ROCHELLE FRIEDMAN
BONNIE GRADSTEIN

Contents

Introduction

Despite medical advances, every pregnancy does not produce a healthy child. Things can and do go wrong. Unfortunately, about one in five pregnancies is lost: approximately one in five women suffers a miscarriage, one in eighty pregnancies ends in the birth of a stillborn child, and one to two percent of all pregnancies are ectopic. About one million women a year in this country have an unsuccessful pregnancy.

The loss of a baby is almost always unforeseen. Although pregnancy loss is not uncommon, it is understandable that pregnant women most often choose not to focus on the possibility. It is a frightening possibility, one that is safer to keep below the surface, in the back of one's mind. "Why should I worry about something that probably will not happen?" is a common reaction. Therefore, when it does happen, it usually comes as a shock, and the woman is unprepared for both the physical and the emotional aftermath. Following pregnancy loss, women are often faced with unexplained feelings and find that they have trouble coping with what has happened. They commonly feel that they have nowhere to turn for help.

Surviving Pregnancy Loss is aimed primarily at women who have experienced either miscarriage, stillbirth, or ectopic pregnancy. Its goal is to help women understand the medical and psychological aspects of what has happened to them and how they are feeling about it. To this end, we have included not only a description of what one typically experiences when a pregnancy is lost, but also, wherever possible, up-to-date medical information about each specific type of loss. In addition, we have drawn widely both upon available knowledge about human behavior and on our own clinical experience in order to give a framework for ordering and understanding the experiences. Lastly, we have included concrete suggestions for coping as well as help in planning for the future.

While this book is not written specifically for women who have had voluntary abortions, we recognize that they may experience feelings similar to those of women who have lost desired pregnancies. Particularly relevant are the sections of this book that address the complex feelings of attachment and yearning that often develop even early in pregnancy and the sections that examine the feelings of grief experienced when pregnancy is lost.

Our clinical experience has shaped the contents and organization of this book. We begin with an overview in which we take a look at the feelings a woman is likely to have during and after the loss of a baby. We then describe each type of loss: miscarriage, stillbirth, and ectopic pregnancy. Even though most readers will have already experienced a pregnancy loss, we have found that it is a critical part of the mourning process to relive the experience; thus the book includes, for each type of loss, a description of the physical experience, a discussion about causes, treatment, and recovery, and a personal account: one woman's story. In addition, each chapter describes emotional reactions unique and specific to that loss. The discussion of each loss is likely to stir memories, trigger conversations, and help the woman understand why the impact of her loss was so great. For those women who have experienced the loss of more than one pregnancy, we have also included a chapter on multiple losses.

We go on to describe the effect of the loss on the woman's partner and to present a personal account of one man's experience. The husband's experience is different in many ways from that of his wife. His emotions and behavior are often misunderstood: this can become a source of conflict in the marriage. The effect on the marital relationship of losing a pregnancy is covered in detail, including cautions of pitfalls to avoid and suggestions for coping. We then focus on the impact of the loss on other children and on family and friends.

We conclude with "Planning for the Future," a section that we hope enables the reader to look toward the future; a future that may include the options of trying another pregnancy, choosing to remain childless, or deciding to adopt. This chapter is designed to give the reader specific information about each option as well as to help her decide which alternatives best suit her and her partner.

We have included a lengthy chapter on adoption because we view it as a particularly attractive option for those who are not biologically able to have a child, as well as for those who do not want to risk another disappointment or live with continual uncertainty. Our experience leads us to conclude that if a couple choose to become parents, the future can hold children for them, whether by birth or adoption.

We suggest that you use the book in the following way. We recommend that everyone read the first section, which deals with the emotional impact of losing a baby. If you have experienced one of the three types of loss, we suggest you read the chapter that applies to you. If you have experienced more than one type, you may want to read more than one chapter as well as the section on multiple losses in chapter II.

We encourage you to read any other chapter that interests you. We do not anticipate that every reader will read every chapter. The goal of this book is not just to educate you, but to help you think about your experience and begin putting it into perspective. We suggest you think about the book as a time line. It can facilitate thinking about the past, coping with the present, and looking toward the future. You may choose to read some chapters now and save others for some future time.

Some readers may wonder why we have included chapters on trying again, adoption, and childlessness. The healing process necessarily takes women into the future and these chapters will provide some of the information they are looking for.

We hope this book will be particularly interesting and useful, too, to families and friends close to those who have lost a pregnancy, as well as to professionals such as doctors, midwives, nurses, social workers, members of the clergy, and others who have contact with people affected by this loss. We anticipate that reading this book will heighten their awareness of the impact that losing a pregnancy can have, and that it will enable them to provide needed support and understanding. In addition, we hope that they will recommend this book to those affected, as a means of helping them in their struggle.

1.

The Experience
of Losing a Pregnancy

"If I could want people who haven't lost a pregnancy to know one thing, it would be to know that it is a real loss. It's not just easy like stubbing your toe. It can be physically painful, like labor. It's not just like having your period. It's the death of a child. It doesn't matter that you can have another, although that is not always true. This particular child is gone and will never come again. You will love the baby you adopt or give birth to in the future, but that is not the child whose loss you have a right to mourn."

1. The Emotional Impact

THE NATURE OF THE ATTACHMENT

All of us come to the decision to have children in our own ways. Some of us have looked forward to parenthood since we were children, while others have come to this choice only later in our lives. Some of us have chosen to have children early in our marriages or before starting a career; others have elected to postpone having children until marriage or career were well under way. Whatever the particular path you traveled to come to this decision, it is likely that once it was made, you became emotionally invested in carrying out your goal.

Pregnancy is a time of hopes, fantasy, and preparation for the future. As you eagerly anticipate the arrival of a child, you psychologically prepare yourself for what life will be like. You imagine what it will be like to hold, feed, or bathe a baby; to see his first smile or witness her first step, and you imagine what it will be like to be a parent.

Concrete preparations are also necessary. If childless, you must prepare yourself for a major change in your life-style. If you already have children, you must tell them about the expected arrival of a new brother or sister; in addition, you need to make plans for coping with the added responsibility that another child will bring. Expectant parents may ready themselves for the new baby by moving to a larger home, stopping or cutting back on work, or arranging for child care. Names may be chosen, a nursery readied, and baby clothes and equipment purchased.

Most people experience pregnancy as a major life event. Some see becoming pregnant as "coming of age," as a confirmation of their passage from childhood to adulthood; while others see it as the fulfillment of themselves as men or women. Whatever the symbolic meaning that it may have had for you, it is likely that losing your pregnancy has influenced where you experience yourself to be in the life cycle. Some couples find themselves extremely frustrated by the discrepancy between their wish to be parents, their readiness to be parents and Nature's failure to comply. They feel eager to move on to the next step in their lives and to take on the responsibility of caring for a dependent being, but they are thwarted in their desire.

For many couples, having a baby is part of a larger life plan. Whether their goal was to bring a child into their lives, create a family, carry on a bloodline, or strengthen a relationship, the loss of a pregnancy deprives them of the possibility of achieving their goal this time. This leaves many couples feeling they are in limbo. They have left one life stage behind, and the next seems to be eluding them. It is most likely that the woman will be able to conceive another pregnancy, carry it without difficulty, and deliver a healthy baby. However, as evidenced by their present situation, there are no guarantees. Those who have had difficulty conceiving, who have lost other pregnancies, or who have had their fertility impaired following an ectopic pregnancy may be particularly concerned about ever being able to have the child they want.

Deciding to have a child is the first step in the process of attachment. Initially we are pulled by a fantasy of ourselves as parents, a vision, if the pregnancy is our first, of what life will be like with a child. We might visualize how our lives will change with another child if we already have one or more. When we do become pregnant our dream promises to come true, and we allow ourselves to become even more attached to a vision of a different future and to the child we are carrying.

Pregnancy is a unique state: it is the only time in life when you are carrying another life within you. On a quite literal level you are not living for yourself alone. On a psychological level it is common to experience the child within you both as part of yourself and as a separate being. It is normal and healthy to feel emotionally fused with the baby you are carrying. During pregnancy you become the center of your own private world, guarding the precious life within. Outside matters touch you differently than they did previously. Feeling that the pregnancy is central to your life and that most of your emotional resources are focused on it is also quite normal. In fact, your ability to visualize yourself as a mother and to form an attachment to the child you are carrying is critical to forming a healthy relationship with your child.

In our clinical experience we have found that it is not unusual for women who wanted to be pregnant and who desired to have a child to experience second thoughts or misgivings, once they are pregnant, about what they have gotten themselves into. This observation has been borne out by two studies that examined how women adjust to pregnancy. Both found that it is quite normal to experience some ambivalent feelings about being pregnant. In addition to being an exciting and gratifying experience, pregnancy, particularly a problem pregnancy, can be uncomfortable, stressful, and even, at times, somewhat frightening.

The woman who finds that she does not like some or all aspects of being pregnant may feel guilty. If the pregnancy is successful her negative feelings are eventually minimized, forgotten, or overshadowed by the positive outcome. Such, however, is often not the case if the pregnancy fails. Then the woman may feel that her ambivalent feelings about being pregnant, about having a child, or about being a mother contributed in some way to the unfortunate outcome of her pregnancy.

Sometimes, however, the loss of a pregnancy highlights the other pole of the mother's ambivalence. It is not unusual to find women who, although initially uncertain about whether they wanted to have a child, no longer are so. These individuals find that the experience of being pregnant and losing the pregnancy has helped them discover how much they really want what they have lost.

The bond that a mother forms to her unborn child is unique. Usually you form an attachment to others on the basis of your love of the other's distinct self and because of his or her relationship to you. In pregnancy, you may feel an attachment to a fetus who is not known to you in the usual way that others in your life are known. The pregnant mother brings a lifetime of experience of knowing, loving, and caring for others to this new and unique relationship.

At first her attachment is to a fantasy image of her future child. She loves a hoped for, longed for child. She may imagine what the baby will look like, what sex it will be, and perhaps even give it a name.

As pregnancy progresses, the mother forms an actual acquaintance with her child, not through the usual ways we come to know others in our lives, but through physical sensations: the baby's weight inside her, its contours and movements. As the fetus grows and becomes more active, the mother increasingly experiences it as separate from herself.

At delivery, the mother is physically separated from her child. It is also necessary for her to cope with psychological separateness: her baby is now a unique being and must be loved as separate from herself. When the birth process proceeds normally, the mother loses the child inside her while gaining an "outside" real baby. When pregnancy fails or a stillbirth occurs, there is both the loss of the child the mother had grown to know and love and the loss of the one she imagined it would someday become. In addition, there will be no baby to compensate for the loss of the internally experienced child.

Attachment begins at different times in the pregnancy for different women. Even for the same woman the attachment process is often somewhat different from one pregnancy to another. Commonly women who have already had a successful pregnancy form an attachment to their future child earlier in the next pregnancy than does an inexperienced mother: they trust that being pregnant will lead to having a child. In contrast, women who have had the experience of losing a pregnancy often find themselves holding back on forming an emotional attachment: they may treat pregnancy as a "condition" and may not allow themselves to think about the child inside them, so as to protect themselves from the pain of loss should the pregnancy fail.

THE NATURE OF LOSS

Why is the loss of a pregnancy so painful? How can you mourn someone you never knew, something that the world tells you was not a baby? Your doctor has probably said something like: "It's all for the best — this is nature's way of assuring that only healthy babies are born." He or she has told you that you can try again in a few months. Then, why does it seem as if your entire life has come to a screeching halt? Why the excruciating grief and yearning that you feel?

The grief that you felt and perhaps still feel when your pregnancy was lost is not as puzzling a response as is often thought. Soon after conception the psychological and physiological processes of pregnancy are set into motion. The level of reproductive hormones in your circulation increases greatly, your uterus develops a thick lining to support the growing fetus, and your breasts enlarge in preparation for nursing. The aim of these processes is to prepare both your body and your psyche for your expected child. When a pregnancy is lost this preparation is interrupted, and you are left in a state of physical and emotional readiness for a baby that will never be.

It is possible, and in fact quite common, to experience a great deal of pain after losing a pregnancy that in actuality had no possibility of succeeding, as with an ectopic pregnancy, or with a "blighted ovum," where the severe nature of the genetic defect makes life impossible. How can one form an attachment to something that was really only a small mass of undifferentiated tissue? The answer to this question is central to understanding why you are feeling so much pain, as well to explaining why the loss feels different to you than to anyone else. Early in pregnancy you formed a mental image of the child you were carrying; this image was a composite of your hopes and wishes and maybe also of your fears. Usually this process begins well before anything remotely like a baby is present. Because your feelings for your future child began before there was a child, and because they grew independently of any actual fetal development, they have a life of their own. This does not make them any the less significant — after all, in other areas of life one has hopes and expectations; and one is sorely disappointed when one's dreams are shattered.

Many factors influence how you experience the loss of a pregnancy. Among these are whether or not the pregnancy was consciously desired, whether or not you already have another child, your age, the length of time you have been trying to have a baby, and whether or not you have lost earlier pregnancies.

Also significant is whether you had formed an attachment to

your future child at the time when your pregnancy was lost. Once the bonding process has begun, the loss of your pregnancy is likely to be quite painful. Pain is experienced on many levels. Foremost there is the loss of your beloved child; there are also the frustration of your hopes for yourself, the loss of your pregnancy, and the denial of your wish to be a parent.

If your loss occurred late in pregnancy after you had felt your baby kick and move and had probably heard its heart sounds during visits to your doctor, the sense of loss that you feel is likely to be intense. You have lost a real baby in addition to a dream. With a late loss you grieve for a baby that you have lived with and loved for many months.

In the months following the loss of a pregnancy, people often ask themselves why they are so upset. This is because many of us may be totally unfamiliar with either the kinds of feelings that we are having, or with feelings of such intensity. Moreover, we may be puzzled by our reaction because we don't understand the true nature of the loss we have experienced.

Because you and your future child shared the most intimate of relationships for a period of time, it is likely that the loss of your pregnancy evoked many of the same feelings you have had when a person whom you have loved has died. This is because for you the fetus was a child and the loss of your pregnancy or of your stillborn baby was a death.

The individual who has lost a beloved person usually experiences several stages of grief. Women who have experienced pregnancy loss commonly go through a parallel grief process. Although the internal experience of loss is essentially the same in both situations, mourning following the loss of a pregnancy differs in several ways from that which occurs after a death. When a fetus is lost there is no tangible "outside" person to mourn, and mourning someone who is not physically present is known to be particularly difficult. In addition, because there are no memories and no shared life experiences the loss often has a feeling of unreality about it.

Contributing to this feeling of unreality is the commonly described experience of finding that the attachment one feels toward one's future child may not be shared by anyone else, even one's spouse. There are many reasons why this is so. Especially when the loss has occurred early in the pregnancy, the mother may be the only one who knows that she is pregnant. She alone at this point has an awareness that something special is happening inside her. This awareness makes the pregnancy "real" for her; thus when the pregnancy is lost she knows that she has lost something, while others have a hard time recognizing that anything much has happened.

While a prospective father may share his wife's desire for a child, the fact that the pregnancy is not part of his physical self makes the experience less immediate, and often less real, for him. One consequence is that the father may feel little or no attachment to his future child until late in the pregnancy, or even not until it is born. Consequently, when the pregnancy is lost in the early months, or even later, as with a stillbirth, the father may not yet have formed an attachment to his child, and so may not mourn its passing as intensely.

Friends, relatives, and even your physician may not understand what the loss of your pregnancy means to you. They did not share your experience and so are probably unaware of the depth of your feelings for your yet unborn child. Because they did not experience the attachment that you felt they may not be able to appreciate your pain, or even understand it, so they may be able to offer you little in the way of support. You may be made to feel that your emotional reactions are inappropriate or excessive, or you may be encouraged to bottle up your feelings and behave as if nothing has happened.

Before you are persuaded to write yourself off as hysterical, unstable, or a failure at coping, keep in mind that in our culture most people are uncomfortable with grief: they have difficulty dealing with strong feelings in others and/or tolerating those same feelings in themselves. It is important to remember that it is *their* inability to tolerate strong, painful feelings that is the problem, and that your feelings are a normal reaction to the loss you have suffered.

When we lose a beloved person, society recognizes the appropriateness of grieving and offers us various social rituals which help us cope with the death. We are permitted to grieve and mourn, and often others mourn with us. When a woman loses a pregnancy, she is confronted by a unique dilemma: although she may feel that she has lost something precious, she may receive little support for these feelings. Many women have felt that one of the most painful aspects of losing a pregnancy was that others in their life were unable to appreciate the extent to which they felt bereaved by their loss.

The loss of a pregnancy is a life crisis that is largely ignored by modern society: the fetus is regarded as a nonperson, and its loss as a nonevent. Society denies the importance of what has happened and discourages the expression of grief by letting the woman know that she didn't really lose anything; she can always try again soon.

GRIEF AND MOURNING

Some women experience severe grief at the loss of a pregnancy; others feel disappointment that is less marked. It is not unusual to mourn for weeks or months after losing a pregnancy or having a stillborn child. It is important to remember that mourning is a slow, painful, but important process of coping with loss. It is not only acceptable to grieve; grieving must take place before healing can occur.

Although not everyone reacts to loss in the way you do, there are some aspects of mourning that are commonly experienced. The initial stage of the grief process is frequently one of emotional numbness and disbelief. Gradually, the full impact of what has happened sinks in, and numbness gives way to a period of active mourning, which may last anywhere from several weeks to many months. During this period one is apt to feel sad, emotionally unstable and somewhat irritable; may cry easily and at the slightest provocation; may be preoccupied with the loss and uninterested in the outside world, and may prefer to avoid contact with anyone or anything that reminds one of the loss. Contrary to popular expectations, a woman probably won't bounce right back and be herself again: healing takes much longer than one might anticipate. Finally the pain lessens and one is able to go on with life.

Each person must progress through the mourning process in his or her own way. How you experience and express grief in pregnancy loss is determined by many factors, including how you usually handle feelings, how you characteristically deal with stress, whether or not you have experienced other losses, how supportive your spouse is, how your social network reacts, what else is going on in your life at the time, and what your prognosis for future success in childbearing is.

Also important are the actual circumstances of your loss. Shock may be particularly severe if you were suddenly confronted by the knowledge that your pregnancy was doomed or that your child had died. Likewise, if you were physically exhausted from labor, the initial impact of the loss may have been overwhelming. Possibly there were indications all along that the pregnancy was in trouble. If this was the case for you, it is likely that you had prepared yourself for the possibility that there might be difficulty and had begun to grieve in advance.

It is not unusual for mourners to deny the death for a brief period of time. It seems too much for them to comprehend and they feel emotionally frozen, apathetic, or confused: reactions that indicate that they cannot deal with the loss at present. When fetal death is diagnosed before labor begins, the couple may still hope that the doctor is wrong, that somehow the baby is alive. Even after the delivery, the parents may continue to deny the death for a brief time.

Nancy, in her late twenties, said: "I had been so happy with my pregnancy — I enjoyed growing big and feeling the baby move. After the delivery of our stillborn daughter, I felt strange. The baby I carried for eight months, who was so much a part of me, my life, my thoughts, was gone. I felt so empty. The first day I kept touching my stomach, I guess to help me feel through my sense of touch, that it was real — my baby was gone. I cried that day but mostly felt numb."

As the reality of the death sinks in, it is common to experience feelings of disappointment, sadness, and yearning. The emotional pain that you feel may be so intense that it feels like a physical sensation: tightness in your chest, a knot in the pit of your stomach, or a feeling of being empty inside. Initially you may not be able to stop crying. Tears may flow continuously, or the pain may come in waves. The sadness that you feel seems to emerge from deep within you, and the tears that flow down your face and the sobs that escape from your throat seem to have bubbled up from a place within you that you didn't know existed. It is not unusual to feel preoccupied with thoughts of one's lost child, and isolated from the rest of the world by grief. For a while, one feels like an observer, a wooden doll who goes through the motions of living but feels nothing.

You may develop specific fears or feel generally anxious. Life feels very fragile after a loss, and it is sometimes difficult to prevent one's concern from spreading. You may fear for your own well-being, your husband's, your parents', or that of other children. For a while it may feel as if danger is everywhere, and as if no one you love is ever safe.

Intense sadness or depression may be accompanied by physical symptoms such as fatigue, listlessness, inability to concentrate, loss of appetite, and difficulty in sleeping. You may feel as if you have no energy, as if the smallest effort is too much for you. Since you don't feel like doing anything for a while, you sit in a chair or lie in bed for hours at a time. Sometimes entire days may slip by that way. You may find that you eat only because others tell you to. Food has no taste, and swallowing is hard because you have a lump in your throat.

You may find yourself unable to take pleasure in people, things or activities that you previously enjoyed, and you may find that you prefer being alone to being with other people. Nothing seems to help, no one understands, and everyone says either too little or the wrong thing. Worst of all, your mind keeps returning to your loss: you review everything that happened and reexperience all of the pain all over again. You find yourself trying to figure out why it happened, and you try first one explanation, then another, then another.

At first everything is a reminder, a song on the radio, babies on television commercials, babies smiling up at you from the pages of every magazine and newspaper. It seems as if pregnant women are everywhere, as if everyone you know is either pregnant or just had a baby.

Often bedtime is the worst time of all. You may experience difficulty falling asleep and difficulty staying asleep. It seems to take you hours to fall asleep; then when you finally manage to doze off you are able to sleep only briefly and fitfully. Frequently women remark that their sleep is disturbed by nightmares. Sometimes the nightmare returns night after night, as was Margery's experience: "I had a terrible recurring nightmare for a year in which the fetus wasn't really dead but was stuck in a bottle of formaldehyde in a closet in the hospital. It was crying, 'Mommy, Mommy, I'm here. Come and get me.' I kept running down the halls, opening closets, and could never find it, even though I saw it in my mind."

For a while your emotions may be so intense, so painful, and so frightening that you may think you will never feel anything else; you may even fear that you are losing your mind. Rest assured; as time passes the pain will gradually fade and you will begin to feel better. However, don't anticipate that the climb back will be a steady one. More often, the months after losing a pregnancy are something like a ride on a roller coaster. You may find that after an initial period during which you experience an unremitting depression, your moods seem to fluctuate widely; one moment you are feeling pretty good; the next, you are in the depths of despair. While normally it takes quite a lot to throw you off balance, in the months following your loss almost anything can destroy your fragile sense of control. Any small thing can trigger the pain all over again. Sometimes you will be aware of what precipitated it; on other occasions you might find that you have plummeted back into a depression for no obvious reason.

In addition to feelings of grief, bereaved people may find themselves having a variety of other painful and perplexing emotions. You may find that you feel unusually irritable and upset by things. Some women report an unusually low tolerance level, while others feel themselves oversensitive to real or imaginary slights. You may discover that you react irritably or with anger to incidents that would not ordinarily bother you and, although you are aware that your reactions are irrational, you are unable to stop yourself. Chances are that you are feeling as if something outside you has taken over your formerly reasonable self. In fact, one probably significant impact on the way you are feeling is that you are experiencing hormone withdrawal. In all likelihood, the level of progesterone in a woman's circulation drops markedly anywhere from several weeks to a few days before the pregnancy is actually lost. Although there is not complete agreement, many physicians feel that the rapid decrease in reproductive hormone levels following the end of pregnancy may be responsible for causing alterations in mood, including a predisposition to depression, anxiety, and irritability.

Unfortunately, this physiological stress hits you at a time when you are both physically and emotionally vulnerable, and so already compromised in your ability to cope. One result of this stress overload is to overtax your normal coping mechanisms, leaving you feeling helpless, out of control, and overwhelmed. When this happens, you may well rely on more primitive or infantile ways of dealing with the world than is usual for you, anger being one such way. It seems as if there is an unhappy coincidence of events — the actual loss of the pregnancy, reproductive hormone withdrawal, and stress overload — all of which are apt to leave you with an unusually low threshold for feeling angry.

One woman commented, "I felt numb, depressed, angry, upset and shaky, and disoriented until I got home. At home, I felt numb, tired, and angry for a few months. I felt many times 'How could this happen to me?' "

The most likely recipients of your anger are those whom you are close to — your spouse, friends, relatives, your obstetrician, or even God. You may be feeling angry with them for things that they did or didn't do, or your anger with them may be more generalized. Your tendency to be easily irritated may lead you to magnify insults, or to misinterpret well-intentioned behavior.

The anger that you feel toward others may also stem from sources other than your irritable state. Sometimes the anger that you feel toward other people in your life results from a projection or a displacement of your own feelings onto them, as when you end up blaming your obstetrician for something that was out of his control. This is not to imply that all the anger you feel is irrational. It is quite probable that you will run into people who minimize your loss and others who treat you in a thoughtless or insensitive manner.

Feelings of guilt often torment both parents. Most people find it difficult to cope with events that are beyond their control and that they do not understand. We are used to living in a world where things happen for a specific reason. However, if you are among the vast majority of couples who have lost a pregnancy, it is likely that the cause of your loss either was not sought, or, if sought, could not be determined. You probably have been unable to learn very much about what happened to you, and you may have had to rely on your fantasies about what might have gone wrong.

In their search for a plausible explanation, many couples find that they keep reviewing the period of the pregnancy before the onset of difficulty for evidence of something that may have gone wrong or that they may have done wrong. A related preoccupation may be reviewing the pregnancy to see possible missed opportunities for preventing the loss. As one woman said, "It is hard to feel that there isn't a reason. I know that the fetus was possibly abnormal, but I still keep on thinking about whether I did anything to cause my miscarriage."

In some cases couples carry a burden of guilt related to a past event: a previous therapeutic abortion, premarital sex, promiscuity, an extramarital affair, or even to sexual practices or fantasies. Sometimes one or both partners may feel guilty for feeling ambivalent about the pregnancy. They may blame themselves for causing their own difficulties and feel that the failure of the pregnancy was a punishment to teach them a lesson.

Annette, a teacher, commented, "I tried to figure out what I did to cause it. Was I too tense during the pregnancy; was that it? Did I eat right? Did I do too much? Was I too sexually active? The doctor would give me no answers."

Many couples find that their own tendency to search for causes and to blame themselves is reinforced by much of society's mythology about pregnancy loss. Everyone has a theory about what may have caused your difficulties. Usually, the theory is shared in the hopes that you will be able to make use of the information and do things differently next time. Nevertheless, it is sometimes difficult to avoid feeling that you are being blamed and to keep from holding yourself responsible.

Patricia found her own way to cope. "When someone makes a comment, I usually say something like, 'If the fetus could not take the stress of everyday living, it was not meant to survive.' I read that in a book and memorized it. I have no intentions of spending the entire nine months of my next pregnancy (see how optimistic I am?) flat on my back, which some have suggested. If someone persists, I intend to say calmly, 'Are you trying to make me feel guilty?' "

The endless cycle of uncertainty, blame, and guilt can be exhausting. Couples who get trapped in this cycle do so because they devote themselves to resolving the uncertainty by searching for an explanation of what happened. Because this is unlikely to be fruitful, their anxiety grows and their need to know what happened may increase even more.

Fortunately, there are several ways out of this predicament. The simplest solution is to come to terms with the unhappy reality that there are things in life that *are* beyond your control. Easily said, but hard to accept. While you are struggling with this issue, it may be useful to think about what you can do to decrease the anxiety that you feel. Several things that others have found helpful are finding a supportive, caring physician, speaking to other women who have lost pregnancies, and sharing their feelings with their husbands. Discussions with such people about real and mythical causes of pregnancy loss should be helpful in alleviating your own concerns.

A reaction that may surprise and dismay you is your envy of women who have children or who are pregnant. It is not unsual for women who have lost a pregnancy to feel singled out by fate and envious of others who appear to be more fortunate. Many women with whom we have spoken have found that they were unable to see a pregnant woman without feeling acutely jealous. More than one woman told of being warned by her husband when a pregnant woman was approaching on the street, so that she could avert her gaze, and so avoid bursting into tears. As one woman said: "It's not exactly that I want what they have; it's just that I want to have a baby too, and sometimes the wanting is so painful that I can't stand it."

Many women find it extremely upsetting to learn that friends or relatives have become pregnant or that they have delivered healthy babies. One woman said: "I wanted to be big and swollen and instead I was empty. My sister-in-law was pregnant and I didn't want to see her. My husband's family said practically nothing about our stillbirth, but my mother-in-law would give me progress reports on my sister-in-law's pregnancy. Her insensitivity hurt me deeply. And I was envious and bitter at my sister-in-law's healthy pregnancy."

Judy, a pretty dark-haired woman who miscarried in the third month of pregnancy for the second time, found herself hating all of her pregnant friends. "I felt so awful about the way that I felt; I was so filled with sadness, jealousy, and anger. I even wished that my best friend, who had become pregnant at about the same time that I did, would miscarry, too. I just couldn't stand to see her afterwards, even though she was empathetic and tried her best to be helpful to me. I just hated her because she had what I wanted and that was that. I know it was irrational, but that's how I felt."

If being with pregnant women or with couples who have small children is very painful, you may want to avoid these encounters for a while. Most people will understand if you explain to them why you are not able to speak to them by phone or be with them for now. A simple explanation should suffice such as: since you lost your pregnancy it has been difficult for you to have contact with anyone or anything that reminds you of your loss.

In the aftermath of losing a pregnancy, some women experience feelings of inadequacy. Many women with whom we have spoken have expressed concerns about their femininity, their bodily functioning, and their capacity to have children. They see other women as competent and complete while they see themselves as inadequate and damaged. They see their failure to produce a healthy baby as evidence of their failure as women.

A woman who had such feelings said, "I had a very difficult time letting friends know that I had a miscarrige. I was embarrassed. I seemed to think I had failed and that other people's knowing about it would make me ashamed. I also hated myself and my body. I thought my body had betrayed me and I could not trust it anymore. This terrible feeling still bothers me."

An often-encountered manifestation of these concerns is the anxiety that many women experience about their ability to become pregnant again. This anxiety is understandable in the case of women who have previously had difficulty conceiving. However, it is not unusual for women who have not had this problem to worry about whether they will be able to get pregnant again.

"Mentally, I was becoming obsessed with conception," Joyce

said. "I was not really interested in much else. I gradually began to believe we would never have children, but I couldn't quit trying month after month."

Not uncommonly, this concern becomes increasingly intense as attempts to conceive again are not met with success. Eileen started to try to conceive again after her third normal menstrual period. Even though she had conceived her first pregnancy in the first month of trying, she was doubtful of her ability to become pregnant again. As several months passed and she still was not pregnant, her concern reached panic proportions and she sought counseling help. Eileen described how in the months since her miscarriage becoming pregnant again had become the focus of her life. "I lived by my basal temperature chart. We had intercourse at the prescribed times even when we didn't feel like it and even if it meant that my husband had to make up an excuse to get out of going out of town. As the end of my cycle neared, my anxiety mounted. It got so that I could not think of anything else. I would go into the bathroom every hour or so to see if I had started bleeding. I interpreted every twitch of pain in my pelvis as either a good omen or a bad one, depending on my mood. I stared endlessly at my chart in an attempt to divine which way the line would be going next. Needless to say, I was not much fun to live with during all of this. Sometimes I wonder how my husband put up with me. The worst time was usually the first day of my period. Then everything looked hopeless. I was sure that there was something wrong with me and I was convinced that I would never have a child."

Most women regard the renewal of their menstrual cycle in the months following their miscarriages as evidence that their bodies have returned to normal. But, like Eileen, those anxious to conceive again often find themselves sad and disappointed with a renewed sense of personal failure with each subsequent period. For many, menstruation is seen as painful evidence of their nonpregnant state, a symbol of their inadequacy and either consciously or unconsciously associated with the lost pregnancy.

A sense of inadequacy may spread beyond the realm of biological functioning for some women. They experience the loss as evidence of their more generalized inferiority and worthlessness. Feelings of inadequacy, loss of attractiveness, physical inferiority, and lack of productiveness can overshadow their previously sound sense of self-worth. A woman who went through this said, "I felt my body was inadequate, inferior, that there was something wrong with it. My husband's disappointment over our loss made me feel I had let him down. The stillbirth colored my whole view of myself. I was negative about myself — I felt worthless, incompetent. From being an outgoing, happy young woman, I became sullen and withdrawn. It took time to build up my confidence again, but I gradually did, with help from my husband."

COPING

In the months following the loss of your pregnancy, some uncomfortable confrontations may be in store for you. Other women who have survived this difficult time have offered suggestions about how to manage.

First, because a nursery full of baby clothes and furnishings may trigger painful feelings, many couples prefer to pack these things away. Others may leave everything as it is in the hope that they will eventually have a baby. You may decide that you would prefer someone else to pack away the baby things before you arrive home from the hospital. On the other hand, doing this yourself may be a way to mourn your loss, or a way to grasp the reality and finality of it. You may want your husband, a family member, or a friend to tell others the bad news for you, or you may want to let people know by yourself. In either case, be prepared to face questions from people who haven't heard. Acquaintances who are unaware of your experience may ask such questions as "How old is your baby now?" "Was it a girl or a boy?" or they may offer congratulations. You may wish to rehearse how you will handle telling your bad news. Although you will probably feel sad each time this happens, you may also find that others can offer you comfort, understanding, and support.

"It was helpful to have people to talk to. I hated being alone. Everyone's obvious sympathy really helped me a lot. No one made light of my grief — no platitudes about how I'd have a baby soon. Instead, more of 'This must be very hard for you.' At home, my friends who'd had miscarriages were great. They really understood the most. One friend who visited started to cry. I cried. We talked and cried for about two hours. When she left, I felt great."

There are certain times, places, events, and people that are certain to be difficult to confront for a while. As we've said, anything even remotely connected with either pregnancy or babies is bound to trigger painful feelings. This may cause otherwise dauntless souls to avoid supermarkets, department stores, parks, or wherever mothers and babies are likely to be. Baby showers, christenings, or first birthday parties are sure-fire reminders. "Don't go to baby showers and pretend to enjoy it — you torture yourself and embarrass others," advises a woman who lost her baby in her eighth month.

Although you can't avoid all uncomfortable situations it is often possible to avoid those that you can anticipate will be painful. Alternatively, some women believe that facing those things that make them uncomfortable is necessary and even hastens the healing process.

Expect to feel waves of sadness return when you visit your obstetrician's office for a postpartum checkup. This was the place where you went in happier times, and also, perhaps, where you learned the bad news. Several women reported that their postpartum visit to the obstetrician's office was very upsetting, and, as one said, "I absolutely hated sitting around the waiting room at my checkup, with all those pregnant women. I don't know how else this could have been handled from the doctor's point of view, but it certainly was no fun sitting there, especially with all the baby care magazines all around."

Some women suggest calling ahead before the visit to request being seen on a day normally reserved for gynecology patients, or requesting the first appointment in a session so as not to have to sit in a waiting room filled with pregnant women. Another suggestion is to inform office nurses and staff of the loss so as to avoid uncomfortable questions about how the baby is doing. If at all possible, have your husband accompany you for your first postpartum visit. He will want to hear what the doctor has to say and he will probably have questions he would like answered. Further, he can be a source of support to you during this predictably difficult time. Think about taking along a close friend or a family member if your spouse is not available.

It is important that you discuss all of your questions and all of your concerns with your physician. Although you may be tempted to avoid sharing your feelings about or toward him, it is often helpful to do so. You may feel that he could have done more, that he made a mistake, that he should have been more supportive, or that he did all that he could, but that you let him down. Also, let him know how you are doing emotionally so that he can assess whether counseling or joining a support group might be helpful to you.

One of the things that your physician may want to discuss with you is his or her understanding of what may have caused the loss. If fetal tissue was available for examination by a pathologist, a report of these findings will also be reviewed. Last, he will advise you about planning for future pregnancies. If he feels that it is important to do diagnostic tests or to initiate treatment of some sort before you try to conceive again, this, too, will be discussed.

Activity

Keeping busy is an excellent way to cope as long as you don't use it to avoid dealing with your feelings: "I have a neighbor and dear friend who is a psychiatric nurse. She encouraged me to come over and cry and talk a lot, which probably kept me from having a nervous breakdown or committing suicide. She talked me into getting a job — any job to keep me busy and put me back into the world again — gave me a purpose for getting dressed and looking good. I got a job as a saleslady in a dress store, and it helped. I cried terribly the days I didn't work. Work kept me together."

A second woman commented, "Keeping busy for a while really helped. I devised all sorts of projects. We took a trip. Ultimately, though, the only thing that really helped was facing up to my grief, my depression — sinking to the depths for me . . . and then deciding I was tired of being unhappy. It was time to get on with life. This took about ten months altogether."

Seeking Help

Normally grief gradually diminishes as time passes, as we have said. When this does not occur you have reason to be concerned that mourning is not progressing as it should. The persistence of denial, of symptoms of depression (sleep difficulty, loss of appetite, irritability, crying, fatigue, or of intense feelings of guilt, anger, blame, or worthlessness) is an indication that you might be having difficulty resolving your grief. Another is the persistence of psychosomatic symptoms (headache, unexplained pain, stomach upset, to name a few) or of self-destructive thoughts or behavior.

Most women find that the loss of a pregnancy or the death of a child is one of life's most agonizing experiences. You are not a failure if you have difficulty coping with the pain. If the pain feels unbearable, or if any of the warning signs just mentioned are present, you should consider seeking help. Increasingly, both professionals and women's support groups are becoming aware that women who have lost a pregnancy or delivered a stillborn child need and deserve such help. Resources are available locally in many communities through clinics and support groups.

Many couples have found that it is very helpful to talk with others who have lost a pregnancy. Since they have been through a similar experience, they know what your loss has been like. They may be able to offer you advice, consolation, and needed support. "Talk to other people who have lost a baby — suddenly they are everywhere," says a young woman, Debbie. "Believe me, they'll more than balance all those 'Oh, don't worry, you'll have another' comments that you are bound to get. Let people know that you have lost something important. Don't keep it bottled up inside."

You might want to join a support group for parents like yourself, or you may even want to organize one. Those who have taken part in such groups claim that the experience of being in a group with people who intuitively know what they had been through was greatly beneficial to them. Among the benefits that membership offered were being able to learn firsthand about how others coped, sharing experiences and feelings, and being able to help others. (For support resources, see appendix.)

Individual psychotherapy or counseling is another route people take to help them cope with their grief. After losing her baby during labor, Christine offered this comment: "Counseling helped me see that my reaction to the death of the child I had envisioned so clearly was not abnormal or overly strong. The pain and shock I felt was normal and experienced by many."

Another woman described her experience: "In counseling I could look forward to releasing my feelings without bugging my friends and husband, all of whom were getting tired of the subject. I definitely got better during this period, but whether it was because of the counseling or because I'd hit rock bottom and was determined to get over my depression, I don't know. Probably some of each. The counseling did give me some insights into why this particular matter had hit me so hard when generally I cope well with problems. Those insights made me feel better about myself — they lessened my guilt about not coping better."

"Counseling showed me I was still a woman," Dorothy, a soft-spoken and attractive red-haired woman, said, "and no less of one because of being unable to have children. It made me look at myself through different eyes. I think counseling helped me to deal with the unexpected emptiness."

How do you decide if you need counseling? Ask yourself if you are able to cope with your emotions. You may need counseling if you have overwhelming feelings of depression, anger or hopelessness, or are feeling so incapacitated by your feelings that you are unable to function.

Planning Another Pregnancy

One way of resolving your loss is by planning for future parenthood, either by trying to get pregnant again or by pursuing adoption.

Before trying to conceive again, you should discuss with your doctor what would be a reasonable waiting period. Your body and your emotions need time to recover. Another pregnancy may simply raise your hopes, anxieties, and tensions before you are ready to deal with them.

You may want to meet with your physician to discuss the cause of death and to obtain a prognosis for future pregnancies. If you were dissatisfied with any aspect of the care you received, talk over your grievances with your doctor. If they can't be resolved, consider changing physicians.

"Find the best medical specialist you can — one who treats you like a human being," a social worker suggested. "I did, and it made all the difference in the world. I had total confidence in my doctor and felt like he really cared for me as a person. That meant a great deal to me."

Those who have experienced the loss of more than one pregnancy or have a history of infertility might consider consulting with an infertility specialist and/or a specialist in high-risk pregnancy.

SUMMARY

It is likely that your life has been significantly altered both by the pregnancy and by the loss you have experienced. Losing a baby may have been your first confrontation with death, your first realization that some events in life are out of your control. Feelings of depression, anxiety, and hopelessness arise not only from the immediate loss, but from an awareness that nothing in life is certain.

This view was expressed by a woman named Janet: "My miscarriage and infertility problems had a great effect on me. While it was a very difficult time, I believe I learned a great deal about myself and about other people. I also learned how important family and children are to me. I learned that I could not cope well with all crises. Previous to this I had always assumed I could handle whatever came my way. I am a deeper, more thoughtful, and more sympathetic person than before. I did not dislike myself before, but I like the 'new me' better. I also fully understand that events in life control us to a far greater extent than I had previously realized. I am more prepared for what life may now deal me. I realize I cannot totally control my destiny."

Grief is a painful fact of life. Fully experienced, it offers one the opportunity to expand one's consciousness, to grow, and to share with family and friends. Stoicism may be greatly admired by some, but only by grappling with grief can one eventually be free of it.

Normally grief gradually diminishes as time passes. However, even when it seems as if the worst pain is finally over, you may find that, on occasion, you still experience periods of sadness, distress and yearning. Sometimes these feelings appear to rise out of the blue: sometimes they are triggered by some painful reminder. As with any loss, even years later you will feel some pain when you remember your loss. The anniversary of your child's death, encounters with children born at about the time that your child would have been: all can reawaken the pain.

It is important to remember that one does not easily get over a loss of the dimension that you have experienced. Mourning takes time. There is no one cure for the pain you feel. Even if you conceive and deliver a healthy baby, it will not erase the loss from your mind. Although the pain diminishes, there will always be reminders, and there will always be the loss of what could have been.

II.

Types of Loss

2. Miscarriage —
An Unrecognized Loss

Susan, a thirty-year-old teacher, and Mike, three years older, were elated when a test showed that Susan was pregnant after six months of trying to conceive. Ten days after the test, Susan began spotting and called her physician. After a pelvic examination, the doctor advised: "Take it easy and let's wait and see. You can continue with your normal routine, but rest as much as you can." For two weeks, she worked only part-time, living in dread that she would lose the baby they wanted so much. Their hopes and excitement over the pregnancy turned to worry when, one evening, the bleeding changed to a red, heavy flow and Susan began to experience intense pelvic pain. Mike rushed her to the emergency room of a hospital, to be met there by her doctor. An hour later, she delivered fetal tissue. Her doctor scheduled a D and C (dilation and curettage) for the next morning to remove from the uterus anything of the pregnancy tissue that might remain. Susan and Mike were shocked at the terrible physical and emotional trauma they had been through during those three weeks. They asked themselves: "How could this happen to two healthy people? What went wrong?"

Although most women know other women who have miscarried, few tend to think about it very much until it happens to them. Susan later reflected: "I now know that miscarriage is fairly common and that it can happen to anyone. Why hadn't I ever heard of it happening to anyone until my miscarriage?"

Because the current United States rates of maternal and infant death are low, it is common for a couple to interpret a positive pregnancy test as a virtual guarantee that they will have a baby at the end of nine months. Susan said: "I suspect if I'd heard more about miscarriage when I was growing up, it might be easier to deal with, but my whole impression was a pregnancy equals a baby, which just isn't so for some of us."

Miscarriage is defined as the spontaneous or natural termination of a pregnancy prior to the twentieth week of gestation. Most couples who have experienced a miscarriage (or spontaneous abortion, as it is also called) are surprised to learn that it is not an unusual event. Few are aware that at least one in five pregnancies ends this way. In fact, the real incidence of miscarriage is even higher than these figures indicate, because statistics do not record those recognized miscarriages that do not come to a physician's attention, or those that go unrecognized and are noted only as delayed or unusually heavy menstrual periods.

With at least a 20 percent chance of miscarriage, why aren't couples aware of this possibility? For one thing, many doctors do not discuss the risk of miscarriage with their obstetric patients. When asked why not, they answer with some variation on "Most pregnancies turn out well, so why should I interfere with my patients' happiness and cause them to worry about something that probably won't happen?" This response indicates that even physicians, aware of the statistical risk of miscarriage, experience difficulty acknowledging that pregnancy sometimes ends in death rather than life. When miscarriage does occur, most couples are totally unprepared. They think of it as the kind of thing that just doesn't happen.

WARNING SIGNS

Women who miscarry usually have some previous warning. Depending on how advanced the pregnancy is, there are a number of signs and symptoms: vaginal bleeding, pelvic pain, no longer "feeling pregnant," and cessation of fetal movement or heartbeat. A fairly typical miscarriage begins with dark brown or red staining lasting several days, which may be accompanied by low abdominal pain and/or backache. This is followed by cramplike abdominal pain and heavy bleeding, and eventually by the passage of fetal and placental tissue.

Vaginal Bleeding

About 20 percent of pregnant women experience vaginal bleeding during the first twenty weeks of pregnancy. Half of these pregnancies will terminate in miscarriage, while the others will reach term successfully. Since it is initially impossible to determine when bleeding will result in miscarriage, most physicians consider any bleeding in early pregnancy a sign of "threatened abortion" or miscarriage.

A doctor should be consulted whenever vaginal bleeding occurs during pregnancy. The seepage may be dark brown, which indicates old blood, or bright red, a sign of more active bleeding. Often the doctor will recommend a pelvic examination to determine if the cervix is closed (an indication that active labor has not begun). He will also try to find the cause of the bleeding. Besides a threatened miscarriage, other causes of vaginal bleeding include ectopic pregnancy, cervical erosions and polyps, and implantation bleeding.

If bleeding is slight or short-lived, the physician probably would decide to wait and see before ordering diagnostic tests. However, persistent bleeding usually warrants a more thorough assessment of the situation.

Pelvic Pain

Cramplike low abdominal pain usually accompanies the bleeding and increases in intensity as the process continues. If a pelvic examination is carried out at this time, it will reveal that the cervix has begun to shorten and dilate, forewarning in most cases the beginning of labor and the inevitability of miscarriage.

Absence or Disappearance of Signs and Symptoms of Pregnancy

Many women experience symptoms such as morning sickness, fatigue, and breast engorgement during the first trimester. A number of women who miscarry either fail to have such symptoms of pregnancy at all or, having had them, notice that they have stopped. In the latter case, bleeding commonly starts several days later.

For some women, the onset of miscarriage is heralded by a vague sense that something is wrong. It is not uncommon for a woman to feel less pregnant and wonder if her breasts are less full, if her abdomen looks less protuberant, or if her queasiness and fatigue have suddenly decreased. These physical sensations can be accompanied by a strange kind of tension and general feelings of dread.

Depending on what warning signs are present, the outcome of the pregnancy may either be known immediately or unclear for a while, at least. The eventual outcome may be unclear when such symptoms as vaginal bleeding, pelvic heaviness, or an apparent decrease in nausea, breast engorgement, or fatigue are present. The symptoms of a threatened miscarriage can persist for anywhere from a few hours to days, weeks, or even months before they cease or miscarriage occurs.

The absence of a previously present heartbeat is an absolute sign of fetal death. Likewise, if the woman's subjective sense that fetal movement has ceased for more than twenty-four hours is confirmed by the examining physician, fetal death may be diagnosed soon after the first warning signs were noted.

Sometimes it is possible to determine the probable outcome of a "threatened miscarriage" using a variety of diagnostic tests. When a woman conceives, a hormone, human chorionic gonadotropin (HCG), produced by the fetal trophoblast (the placenta) may be detected in the mother's urine or blood. Measurement of the beta subunit fraction of HCG can let your doctor know if the fetal placenta is still functioning and whether the fetus is still alive. (This is a more sensitive test than a routine pregnancy test.) Another procedure, the diagnostic ultrasound, can also be used to assess whether the fetus appears to be viable. This test uses sound waves to form a picture, and in this way can demonstrate whether an embryonic sac and a fetus are present, indicating that the pregnancy is still viable. Likewise, if the pregnancy is sufficiently advanced for a fetal heartbeat to be present, ultrasound examination will reveal if one can be found, thereby determining whether the fetus is dead or alive.

COPING WITH THE SIGNS OF MISCARRIAGE

Women respond differently to the first signs of difficulty. Some feel an immediate sense of panic and dread, others feel concern but remain optimistic, and some feel shocked, disbelieving, and frozen. If the warning signs persist for a prolonged period of time, it is likely that periods of optimism will alternate with times of despair and disbelief. Susan, whose miscarriage was described earlier, tearfully described her feelings of cold dread as she saw that the paper with which she was wiping herself was stained with blood. "I just sat there not believing that this was happening to me. I think that I cried but I don't remember feeling very much. I know that for the next few hours I kept going back into the bathroom to see if there was still blood — each time wishing that it had all been a mistake. When I called my doctor and told him what had happened, he asked me to come over to his office so that he could examine me. I felt totally panicked. When he examined me and found that my cervix was closed and that my uterus seemed to be the right size, I felt a bit relieved, maybe it was not going to be so bad after all. I can hardly remember anything about the next two weeks other than checking to see if I was still bleeding — feeling hopeful when I wasn't, and terror-stricken when I was."

In some ways the most difficult period begins with the first awareness that there may be something wrong. There can be days, weeks, or even months of uncertainty. Reactions to this situation vary. It is not uncommon for a woman to put her feelings about the pregnancy "on hold" as a way of protecting herself against the possibility that it will be lost. Nor is it unusual for her to be obsessed with anxiety and incapable of thinking about anything else.

This period of uncertainty can be a difficult one. Nonetheless, many women feel best about themselves when they try to gain some control over the situation: for instance, informing the physician when any of the above "danger signs" are present. It is tempting to deny the implications of what may be happening — to tell yourself that you are just imagining it. Many women who did told us they remember thinking at the time, "I don't want to disturb my doctor"; "I'm just overreacting — I'll feel like a fool if everything is normal"; and "It's just minor. I'll wait to see what happens." But denying the problem or acting stoically isn't a good idea. Being afraid of bad news is all the more reason to take action, so you can either relax or begin to deal with what may occur. It is better to make a mistake because you're too concerned; waiting too long to seek medical attention can jeopardize the pregnancy, your health, or even your life.

Your physician probably will take your concerns seriously and tell you his initial impression as well as what course of action he plans to follow for the present, or anticipates following in the future if your symptoms either continue as they are or became more severe.

Women who experienced a miscarriage have told us how important the support of husband, family, and friends were to them in the uncertain period. Many found it helpful to share fears and concerns, to have someone accompany them to the doctor's office or to the hospital for diagnostic tests, and to receive help in making whatever decisions needed to be made. Generally it was agreed that the concern and caring of others was helpful in getting them through this very stressful and alarming time.

THE PHYSICAL EXPERIENCE OF MISCARRIAGE

For many women the physical experience of miscarriage is upsetting, even extremely frightening. Often one is unprepared for what an actual miscarriage is apt to be like. In addition, since miscarriage occurs early in pregnancy, most women will not yet have had any formal preparation for labor and delivery. Very early miscarriage, as we have said, may be quite similar to a very heavy menstrual period. In contrast, late miscarriage may follow a course not unlike that of a full-term labor and delivery.

It is important to know that heavy bleeding, with or without the passage of clots or tissue, is an indication of impending miscarriage. Cramping or low abdominal pain and watery discharge from the amniotic sac through the vagina are other common indications.

Sometimes miscarriage follows such a rapid course that it is not possible to get to the doctor's office or to a hospital in time. If this should happen to you, you should, if possible, place fetal tissue, which appears as a grayish red mass or blood clot, in a clean container and bring it along to the hospital for the pathologist to examine.

If the miscarriage occurs while you are in the hospital, the physician will check to see if all of the pregnancy tissue (fetus, placenta, and amniotic sac) have been passed. If it happens at home, he or she will conduct an exam afterward.

If all of the fetal and placental tissue has been expelled, the miscarriage is considered to have been complete. Pain and severe bleeding stop, and usually no further treatment is necessary. However, a blood-stained vaginal discharge, called lochia, may persist for several days, until the site where the fertilized egg had implanted itself in the uterus has healed. "Complete" miscarriage usually occurs before the eighth week of pregnancy and is uncommon later in pregnancy.

When only part of the pregnancy tissue is expelled, the miscarriage is said to be "incomplete." Incomplete miscarriages happen more frequently after the eighth week of pregnancy, after the placenta is more strongly attached to the uterus. In case of incomplete miscarriage, or as a precautionary measure when it is unclear whether all tissue has been passed, it is usual to keep the patient in the hospital.

If the physician is not sure if the miscarriage was complete, he will perform a minor operation known as a D and C, mentioned above, to empty your uterus. During a D and C, the cervix is stretched and a spoon-shaped instrument called a curette is inserted through the cervix and used to scrape the uterus. The procedure is usually performed under anesthesia and in a hospital.

Immediately after spontaneous miscarriage or after a D and C, the uterine muscles contract. This action blocks exposed uterine blood vessels, keeping bleeding to a minimum. When this happens, you may experience abdominal cramps much like menstrual cramps or labor pains. These cramps, or afterpains, are usually most intense right after the delivery of the fetus has occurred. Thereafter, they decrease in intensity and frequency. Some women have afterpains for a day or two following the loss of a pregnancy.

Many women who have had a second-trimester miscarriage have found that on the second to fourth day afterward their breasts became engorged with milk. Since one's body has no way of knowing that the fetus has died, it reflexively prepares for breast feeding. Engorgement may cause some physical discomfort, but normally the actual physical pain is less troublesome than the emotional pain that may accompany it. Usually, engorgement will diminish in a day or two. It is important to refrain from expressing milk to alleviate discomfort, as doing this only leads to an increase in milk production. Aspirin may be taken if there is a great deal of pain. Hot wet compresses or ice packs applied to the breasts can also be used to decrease discomfort.

MISSED ABORTION

In some cases the fetus dies in the uterus, but is not expelled. This miscarriage is then classified as a missed abortion. A missed abortion may occur at any time during the first twenty weeks of pregnancy. Typically, a woman who has a missed abortion has experienced several months of normal pregnancy, with fatigue, enlargement of the uterus, breast fullness, and possible nausea. After the fetus dies, the signs of pregnancy gradually disappear. Commonly, the woman will notice that her breasts are less full, that she no longer experiences nausea, and that she has lost some weight. A brownish vaginal discharge is usually observed, and in more advanced pregnancies fetal movements are no longer felt. Pelvic examination will reveal that not only has the uterus failed to grow, but that it has become smaller and lacks the soft consistency characteristic of pregnancy. Some women with a missed abortion will not have any vaginal discharge or bleeding. Then the presumptive diagnosis is usually based on the absence of normal uterine growth.

If a missed abortion is suspected, the diagnosis of fetal death is usually made following one or more tests. Within several days of the death, placental function usually ceases and human chorionic gonadotropin (HCG) is no longer produced. Urine or blood tests for the level of HCG often read negative (no HCG present) soon after the fetus dies; thus, if a previously positive test becomes negative, it is likely that fetal death has occurred. Sometimes, however, the placenta continues to function for several weeks and the test remains positive. In such cases, ultrasonic examination can demonstrate whether or not the amniotic (fetal) sac is empty, which indicates that no fetus can be detected, or whether a fetal heartbeat is no longer present.

Labor: Spontaneous or Induced?

Once the diagnosis of fetal death is made, there are two possible courses of action: awaiting spontaneous labor, which usually occurs within a few weeks, or having labor induced.

There are no medical advantages to waiting until labor begins spontaneously. In fact, since a potentially life-threatening problem, intravascular coagulation (clotting), can occur when a dead fetus is carried by the mother for more than four weeks after fetal death has occurred, most physicians will allow the pregnancy to be carried no longer than this before suggesting that labor be induced.

Still, some women prefer not to have labor induced immediately. Some who have made this choice have felt that they needed a little time with their baby before they were willing to let it go. Others expressed a need for time to deal with the death, while a number of women preferred that labor and delivery be as natural as possible.

Many women, on the other hand, find that it is very upsetting to carry a dead fetus. Instead, they elect to have labor artificially induced. For those who have suffered through days or weeks of warning signs of an impending miscarriage only to end in fetal death, the decision to have labor induced is a means "to get it over with and go on with life," as one woman put it.

Recently, the use of prostaglandins has made the induction of labor in a woman with a missed abortion safe and reliable.

Georgia and Tom chose to wait for labor to begin naturally after they learned of their baby's death at five months. "We had been reading about natural childbirth and had just begun attending classes in it. We wanted to quickly finish learning about it and continue as we had planned. We felt it would give us some time to adjust to the death. We couldn't believe it at first. And we knew we wanted to try again and the labor and delivery experience would be helpful in a future pregnancy."

The physician usually discusses the pros and cons of both options. However, unless there are overriding medical considerations, the final choice is usually left to the woman.

It is common to feel a resurgence of grief once delivery has taken place, even if mourning took place when fetal death was first diagnosed. This is because at the delivery, secret hopes that the fetus "was really alive in spite of all indications to the contrary" must be finally abandoned.

THE HOSPITAL STAY

If miscarriage occurs prior to the twentieth week of pregnancy and all pregnancy tissue is passed spontaneously, hospitalization may not be necessary. However, if fetal death occurs after the twentieth week, if the miscarriage is incomplete, or if it is not possible to determine whether or not all tissue has been passed, the woman will be admitted to the hospital so that a D and C can be performed, as we have said above. A D and C is done whenever there is a danger that the miscarriage may have been "incomplete," since the failure to remove all pregnancy tissue from the uterus may cause hemorrhage.

Many factors conspire to make the hospital experience a difficult one for the woman who has miscarried. Since the routines in most hospitals are planned around women delivering healthy full-term babies, it is quite likely that many hospital practices and regulations do not meet the miscarrying woman's needs.

Hospitals differ greatly in their treatment of women who have miscarried. The best ones offer a choice of accommodations, helpful and supportive nursing care, and even in-hospital counseling. However, such is not always the case.

Women who were hospitalized told us that the experience was less painful than it might have otherwise been when they were able to arrange the following things:

(1) to have their husbands be with them as much as possible, including during labor, and delivery and in the recovery room; when overnight hospitalization was necessary, some women asked that their husbands be allowed to stay with them;

(2) to be hospitalized on a floor other than the maternity floor;

(3) to have a private, rather than a shared, room if desired;

(4) to discuss in advance with the physician whether to have local or general anesthesia during delivery or during the D and C;

(5) to decide in advance whether or not to see the fetal tissue;

(6) to decide how the fetal tissue would be disposed of.

* * *

(Since hospitalization is an integral part of the stillbirth experience, it is covered in more detail on pages 64–67.)

CAUSES

One of the first questions couples ask after a miscarriage is "What caused the miscarriage to occur?" In many cases, unfortunately, it is not possible for the physician to determine the specific cause, even following pathological examination of fetal tissue. Sometimes it is impossible to determine whether or not there are any abnormalities present. In other situations, one or more potential causes may be found but it is not possible to determine whether one particular factor is, in fact, the significant one. This means that it is quite likely that you will not be able to find out exactly what caused you to miscarry. This is frustrating in and of itself, but doubly troubling in that the failure to determine a cause leaves both you and your physician in the dark about what to look for and what treatments to try in subsequent pregnancies. Reflecting on two miscarriages, Lynn said: "I wish someone could diagnose the *why* of either miscarriage. The worst part is having to go through all that without anyone ever being able to give an explanation."

Abnormal Fetal Development

Medical research has demonstrated that the single most common cause of miscarriage is an abnormality in the development of the egg (the ovum) that is incompatible with life. These pregnancies are destined to fail from the very outset, as the chromosomal or genetic abnormality is too severe to permit the fertilized ovum to survive. When the ovum dies, hormonal support for the pregnancy stops. Sometime after this, the defective ovum is expelled. Since the developmental abnormality in these "blighted" ova is so severe that survival is not possible, there is no treatment that can save the embryo.

Most blighted ova pregnancies result from random factors that are unlikely to be repeated and so do not pose a risk to subsequent pregnancies or to future children. The earlier the miscarriage, the more likely it is that chromosomal factors are responsible.

In accepting her loss, one woman expressed it this way: "I deeply feel that if a miscarriage occurs, there is a reason and it's best to let it go. The baby would have had problems and it's nature's sad but wise way of protecting everyone concerned."

Hormonal Factors

(1) PROGESTERONE It is well known that the reproductive hormones estrogen and progesterone play an active role both in permitting pregnancy to occur and in maintaining pregnancy once conception takes place. What is less well established, however, is what role, if any, progesterone deficiency plays in causing miscarriage.

Research is currently under way studying the effects of progesterone deficiency on the uterine lining (the endometrium) during the postovulatory phase of the menstrual cycle. Investigators have attempted to treat women with an inadequate postovulatory phase (believed to be caused by progesterone deficiency) with progesterone prior to implantation of the fertilized ovum in the hope that miscarriage will be prevented.

Another research project focuses on giving progesterone to women with a well-established pregnancy. These women were considered a high risk because of existing symptoms of "threatened miscarriage" or a previous history of pregnancy loss. This treatment was based on the theory that either the placenta or the corpus luteum might not be producing adequate amounts of progesterone and that the administration of progesterone may be effective in preventing miscarriage.

Unfortunately, to date, neither type of treatment has been definitively demonstrated to be effective. In addition, there is evidence that prenatal exposure to female sex hormones may cause developmental abnormalities in the fetus. For these reasons, most physicians are reluctant to prescribe progesterone for the prevention of miscarriage unless a postovulatory-phase defect can be clearly demonstrated and all other types of treatment have been exhausted.

(2) ENDOCRINE SECRETIONS There is some evidence that disorders of the thyroid or the pituitary gland may in a very few women in-

terfere with their ability to become pregnant and, once they are pregnant, may increase the risk of miscarrying.

Uterine Disorders

Some uterine abnormalities may affect the growth and development of the fetus. A woman may be born with two uterine compartments instead of the usual single chamber. Others may have either an unusually small uterus, or other developmental abnormalities. The presence of one or more large uterine fibroid tumors (benign growths) may also pose a problem.

While both uterine abnormalities and fibroid tumors are associated with an increased risk of miscarriage, not every woman who has these conditions experiences difficulty in carrying a pregnancy to term. If, however, the specific uterine abnormality is such that the fetus does not have room to grow, miscarriage will eventually occur. Surgical correction of uterine structural problems and fibroids offers many women with these problems a good chance for success in subsequent pregnancies.

Cervical Incompetence

An "incompetent" cervix, a cervix that fails to remain closed for the duration of the pregnancy, is still another structural abnormality that may be associated with an increased risk of miscarriage. Why some women have cervical incompetence is not known. In others, it seems to occur secondary to cervical damage sustained during dilation of the cervix for tests, or in the course of traumatic delivery or therapeutic abortion. Characteristically, the woman with an incompetent cervix usually does well during the first trimester of pregnancy. But as the fetus increases in size and weight during the second trimester, the already weakened cervix dilates prematurely, thus threatening the continuation of the pregnancy. Since this dilation occurs in the absence of painful uterine contractions, it often goes unrecognized by the woman and undiagnosed by the physician until the pregnancy is already lost. When diagnosed early, on the other hand, it can be treated by encircling the cervix with stitches or with a band that keeps it closed. This procedure is most often performed some time between the fourteenth and twentieth week of pregnancy. The closure is usually removed by cutting the band or the stitches when it is time for labor.

Cervical incompetence is a relatively rare cause of miscarriage. Only approximately one in a hundred miscarriages occur for this reason. However, it should be considered as a possible cause of miscarriage when the pregnancy is lost between the third and the sixth month. Moreover, women who have had one late miscarriage should be followed closely in subsequent pregnancies for signs of cervical incompetence.

Other Factors That May Cause Miscarriage

(1) BLOOD TYPE INCOMPATIBILITY Controversy exists about whether blood type incompatibility of either the Rh or ABO system in the parents increases the likelihood that early miscarriage will occur. Blood group incompatibility, however, has clearly been demonstrated to contribute to the loss of pregnancy after twenty weeks.

(2) DES EXPOSURE Diethylstilbestrol (DES), a synthetic estrogen, was first used as a medication to prevent fetal loss in 1945. It was used for this purpose until 1971, when an association was discovered between DES exposure and a rare form of vaginal cancer in the daughters of women so treated. There followed shortly the discovery that DES exposure was also associated with unusual but characteristic abnormalities of the vagina and cervix among these daughters. Although it was originally feared that these vaginal and cervical abnormalities might be associated with the later development of vaginal cancer, this concern appears not to have been borne out. Happily, the overall incidence of vaginal cancer in DES daughters is also much lower than was originally predicted.

In recent years, DES exposure has been linked to a variety of fertility problems. Clinical studies have indicated that women whose mothers took DES show a somewhat reduced ability to conceive, compared to the overall population. DES exposure has also been held responsible for a higher than usual incidence of tubal pregnancy. Although as yet the association between DES exposure and both miscarriage and prematurity has not been conclusively established, there is evidence to indicate that women exposed to DES have a higher than average incidence of uterine abnormalities, cervical incompetence, first and second trimester miscarriage, and premature births.

(3) MATERNAL DISEASE An increased rate of fetal loss (miscarriage and stillbirth) has been linked with a number of infectious diseases. Some viral agents are thought to be responsible for both congenital malformations and miscarriage. A higher than normal incidence of both types of difficulty are found in women infected with the following viruses: rubella (German measles), cytomegalovirus, herpes simplex virus, measles, mumps, polio, chicken pox, and hepatitis. Fortunately, these infections tend to be quite uncommon during pregnancy.

T mycoplasma, an infectious agent which has characteristics of both bacteria and viruses, has been found in the tissues of some aborted fetuses. This microorganism has been implicated as a cause of both infertility and of miscarriage. While research studies have not definitively demonstrated that T mycoplasma causes either infertility or miscarriage, since both tests to isolate this agent from the parents and antibiotic treatment are easily obtained and without risk, many physicians treat couples whose cultures are positive. When a positive culture is obtained, both parents are treated with a course of antibiotics (usually tetracycline) prior to attempting another pregnancy.

The risk of miscarrying is somewhat increased for women who have certain chronic illnesses. This is particularly true when the illness is severe. Diabetes, systemic lupus erythematosis, some heart conditions, kidney disease, and markedly elevated blood pressure, are all associated with an increased rate of miscarriage.

(4) RADIATION EXPOSURE Exposure to significant amounts of ionizing radiation has been linked with both an increased incidence of miscarriage and an increased incidence of congenital malformations. Exposure to all types of X rays should be avoided during pregnancy unless absolutely necessary. If at all possible, ultrasound, which uses high-frequency sound waves, should be used in preference to diagnostic X rays during pregnancy.

(5) MALNUTRITION While poor nutrition has been implicated in many complications of pregnancy, the role of vitamin and protein deficiency in causing miscarriage has never been conclusively proven.

(6) MATERNAL AGE The risk of fetal loss of all types, including miscarriage, is significantly greater for women under the age of twenty and over thirty-five than for women between these ages. Why this is so is not known.

(7) USE OF ALCOHOL The Surgeon General's Advisory on Alcohol and Pregnancy warns that alcohol consumption during pregnancy, especially during the early months has been demonstrated to be harmful to the fetus. An increase in the rate of miscarriage is one of several hazards associated with alcohol use during pregnancy. Women who consume one ounce of absolute alcohol (two standard drinks) twice a week have been reported to experience a significantly increased rate of miscarriage. The effect of lower levels of alcohol consumption or less frequent use carries an as yet unknown risk, as no absolutely safe level of alcohol consumption has been established.

(8) USE OF MARIJUANA The American Medical Association has officially labeled marijuana a dangerous drug. Marijuana use has been demonstrated to affect reproductive function adversely in a variety of ways, including increasing the likelihood that miscarriage will occur. In a study in which female monkeys were treated with THC, the active chemical in marijuana, for three to five years at doses comparable to daily consumption for humans, the miscarriage rate was found to increase significantly.

(9) USE OF TOBACCO Smoking has been implicated in increasing the risk of miscarriage. Although all of the evidence is not yet in, it seems advisable that cigarette smoking should be stopped during pregnancy.

(10) USE OF CAFFEINE There is evidence to indicate that the consumption of caffeine during pregnancy is associated with an increase in the incidence of miscarriage. It is advised that beverages such as coffee, tea, and colas and drugs containing caffeine be eliminated from use during pregnancy.

(11) TRAUMA Only in extremely rare instances are either physical or emotional traumas thought to be responsible for causing miscarriage. Travel by car, train, or plane has not been associated

with an increased incidence of miscarriage. Similarly, most pregnant women can work, exercise in moderation, and engage in sexual intercourse without jeopardy either to themselves or to the fetus. The reason for this is that the fetus is well protected. First, it is surrounded by a pool of amniotic fluid, which acts as a shock absorber, then by the membraneous amniotic sac, and by the muscular wall of the uterus. The mother's visceral organs and, finally, her skin form additional layers of protection. Pregnancy has been known to continue successfully despite serious accidents, major surgery, exhaustion, or emotional stress. In fact, it is doubtful whether anything but the most extreme environmental factors can disrupt a well-established pregnancy.

(12) ENVIRONMENTAL FACTORS Exposure to pesticides and other toxic chemicals should be avoided during pregnancy, as evidence is accumulating to indicate the harmful effect of many of these substances on the developing fetus.

Psychological Factors

When a woman miscarries, she, her husband, family, and physician all seek a tangible reason for why the pregnancy failed. Frequently, none is found. Most couples have a great deal of difficulty dealing with this uncertainty. Every event or occurrence is scrutinized in an attempt to find an explanation for the unexplainable. It is almost as if a "cause" must be found before the miscarriage can be put behind them.

An entire mythology about miscarriage has developed over the years and attests to the strong need to understand what has happened. Most myths imply that a particular activity, event, or psychological experience, one that is deemed of marginal acceptability during pregnancy, is responsible for the miscarriage.

The notion found in traditional psychoanalytic theory that miscarriage may be caused by emotional conflicts is one such myth. Classical theory maintains that miscarriage may be a physical expression of the mother's negative or ambivalent feelings toward either the pregnancy or the mothering role. This theory offers little support to the woman who has miscarried and, in fact, quite clearly blames the victim for bringing her difficulties upon herself.

The research studies and clinical treatment upon which this theory was based were both seriously flawed. It is unfortunate that until the past few years, these flaws were totally overlooked and thus a theory that was decidedly hostile to women was accepted by both the medical establishment and society.

The psychosomatic theory of miscarriage was based upon the clinical studies and treatment of women who had previously experienced one or more miscarriages. According to the investigators, these women were more immature, emotional, and "neurotic" than other women. However, the investigators failed to take into account what these women were like before they had miscarried, since they saw them only after the miscarriage. Most individuals experience the loss of a desired pregnancy as traumatic and have a period of heightened emotionality lasting anywhere from a week or so to several months afterward, so it is not unusual that researchers found the women to be "emotional." There is no real evidence that a woman's emotional state during the pregnancy influences whether or not she will miscarry, or that her emotional state afterward indicates anything meaningful about her emotional state before the loss of the pregnancy.

The utility of psychotherapeutic treatment in reversing a woman's tendency to repeatedly miscarry has been claimed but never actually demonstrated. Nevertheless, the alleged success of this treatment was used by supporters of the psychosomatic theory as evidence supporting their original claims. In sum, there is no solid evidence that supports the notion that emotional factors play a significant role in the causation of miscarriage.

WILL IT EVER HAPPEN AGAIN?

A concern commonly voiced by couples who have suffered a miscarriage is "What are the chances that our next pregnancy will be successful?" If the miscarriage was your first or second, the response to this question is quite encouraging. After one miscarriage, the statistical risk of having a second miscarriage is about the same as the risk of a miscarriage in the first place. In all likelihood, each was caused by random, unrelated events that have little likelihood of recurring.

A woman is said to be a "habitual aborter" if she has had three or more consecutive pregnancies terminating in miscarriage.

Whether each of the miscarriages was caused by random factors, or whether they were caused by a recurrent, underlying difficulty must be assessed for each individual. Habitual abortion will be dealt with more extensively in the chapter "Multiple Losses."

TRYING AGAIN

There is some disagreement among physicians about how long to wait after a miscarriage before trying to conceive again. Ninety percent of women will have their first menstrual period four to six weeks after miscarrying. Some physicians feel that if a woman is anxious to conceive, she can begin trying after her first menstrual period. The more usual view is that the chance of a repeat miscarriage is decreased if she waits until she has had three normal periods before attempting a new pregnancy.

Sexual relations may be resumed when the bleeding has stopped and the cervix is closed, which usually occurs three to four weeks following a miscarriage.

Medical Treatment

Most cases of miscarriage have no discernible cause. The failure to find a cause is usually a good sign, as it indicates that random factors were probably responsible, and that a recurrent difficulty is not present.

Most physicians feel that it is unjustified to perform a comprehensive evaluation after a woman has had one miscarriage, because the odds are in favor of a nonspecific or random cause. Medical evaluation is usually recommended after a woman has miscarried two or three times consecutively. If evaluation reveals a specific cause, treatment will be aimed at dealing with that difficulty.

HORMONAL TREATMENT It is felt to be unjustified as a way of treating miscarriage of unknown cause. Estimates are that progesterone deficiency is involved in only 4 percent of miscarriages. In those cases where it can be demonstrated that the woman has a clear postovulatory-phase insufficiency due to progesterone deficiency, progesterone may be administered soon after conception has occurred. There is no evidence that progesterone is effective in treating "threatened miscarriage" because by the time bleeding has started the pregnancy is usually unsalvageable, since fetal death usually precedes the onset of bleeding by several days or weeks. Since this treatment carries some potential risk to the fetus, it must always be carefully considered.

CHROMOSOMAL ABNORMALITIES These are found in a large percentage of miscarried fetuses. The vast majority of these probably occur secondary to random, nonrepeatable events. Chromosomal study is usually recommended after the miscarriage of two, or more usually three, consecutive pregnancies. If a chromosomal abnormality is found that has a high likelihood of recurring in subsequent pregnancies, genetic counseling is normally suggested.

UTERINE ABNORMALITIES Uterine abnormalities may be diagnosed using a combination of pelvic examination and hysterogram (dye is inserted into the uterus and visualized by X ray). Surgical correction is performed whenever it increases the chance for a successful pregnancy. Conditions that may be corrected surgically in many cases include uterine fibroid tumors, double uterus, and cervical weakness or incompetence.

Screening for Underlying Difficulties
Screening for systemic disease and thyroid gland malfunction may be attempted as part of a complete evaluation, although the likelihood of such screening being fruitful in an otherwise healthy, asymptomatic woman is very small.

One Woman's Story

MARCH 1979
I was unprepared for the unrelenting grief, for the intensity of it. I kept thinking, "What is wrong with me? I should be over this by now. I shouldn't be so obsessed with it all — the maternity shops I go by, the Pampers com-

mercials on television. I should be able to call my pregnant and recently delivered friends without struggling to carefully modulate my voice; without needing to give myself a pep talk before I dial the phone. And yet, I still cry. I cry out of control. I cry over trivia, and over everyday occurrences, and over how alone I feel. I still cling desperately to the hope that THIS month, I will be pregnant again, and be able to feel my belly growing and my breasts filling, and my baby kicking inside. My usual methods for coping with stress have been pretty useless."

I am a psychiatrist, and this somehow made me think that I would be able to handle my feelings rationally. I reasoned that many women go through things like this; I have close friends who have miscarried and I have other friends who have had trouble conceiving. I tell myself that I should be able to get through this without falling apart.

What I have learned in a most painful way was that before this happened to me, I really had no idea of what my friends had to bear. I had been as insensitive and ignorant toward them as I now feel people are to me. It wasn't all my fault, of course. They hadn't really tried to talk with me about what they were going through.

I didn't know before it happened to me that I would begin to wonder if there was something wrong with me, that I couldn't do this natural, simple thing that all other women do, often without even wanting to. Everything was as usual in my life: my work, my son, my home, my husband . . . EVERYTHING . . . except that every minute feels like a year to me, every day takes forever, and all I can think about is loss, death and the damn calendar. Spring is here, and instead of feeling happy, I feel miserable. I thought I would be round and well on my way by now, and instead, my body in its smallness seems a perpetual rebuke and a reminder of what I don't have. For everyone else the winter happened and is over, while I feel suspended in time, waiting, counting until I can be pregnant again.

When I happen, by chance, to see a pregnant woman on the street, I can't control my need to stare. I feel miserably torn between fascination, envy, and rage that it isn't me that is pregnant.

I just wasn't prepared for how awful I feel: the isolation, the gauze wrapping of depression. In contrast to my usual ability to be funny, light, and social, I am unable to be casual or light about anything. I am obsessed with worry that something may be wrong with me; that I will miscarry again; that I'll never have another child.

Sometimes it is comforting to be with my son. At other times I can't tolerate *my love for him, because he reminds me of what I have lost. I don't know why but I worry about his health, my health, my husband's health. I feel a sense of urgency about having another child: I worry that there will be too much space between children, and I worry that I am getting too old. I don't seem to be able to relax, and wait the required months before trying again.*

My second miscarriage was at eleven weeks, and it took about nine days from the time I started with a bit of brownish discharge to the day I miscarried. I've read that most women don't allow themselves to acknowledge the possibility of miscarriage, and so if it happens, it comes as a complete shock. My experience was quite different in that I had misgivings about this pregnancy from the beginning. Perhaps this was because I had had a very early miscarriage four months before; perhaps because I had had a healthy term pregnancy and I knew what it felt like. In any case, I'd had cramps early in the pregnancy and had never felt very pregnant. No nausea, almost no fatigue, few of the subtle physical changes that I had experienced the first time. I found myself continually trying to explain these vague misgivings to my husband and to my obstetrician. I felt that I didn't want to invest too much or tell too many people.

In some ways I was not surprised when I began to have some spotting. I was, nevertheless, intensely upset. I hesitated before checking with my doctor lest he think I was being "hysterical" and "overreacting." I spent four days doing little other than noting every twinge, cramp, and bit of vaginal discharge. On the fifth day I woke up feeling different. Less pregnant, even, than I had felt before. My stomach felt a little bit shrunken, my breasts totally untender.

My husband tried to be reassuring, but his calmness left me feeling isolated. I went to work, not knowing what else to do, because it all seemed so subjective. I tried to go through the day as if everything was fine, but I knew that everything was all wrong.

As I left work that evening and walked to my car, it was snowing. I was concentrating on not moving too fast so I wouldn't have more spotting. I got home; we ate dinner. I stood up to take some dishes to the sink and felt uncomfortably bloated for a moment; then I felt a warm sticky trickle run down my legs, and I ran into the bathroom.

Although I felt a terrible rush of fear, I tried to stay calm, partly so as not to upset my son, and partly to delay the impact of what I knew had happened. Looking at the bright red blood as it flowed into the toilet, I felt surprised to feel all of the things that I had thought I wouldn't experience, because I was psychologically so "well prepared." But they were all there: grief, disappointment, anger, emptiness, isolation, and uncertainty about what to do next. I didn't cry right away. I held myself together beautifully until I had to tell the people I cared about — my husband, my child, my parents and my sister, and a few special friends. With them, I couldn't be brave.

The next four days were a nightmare; perhaps the hardest time in my life so far. The uncertainty was so terrible that it was almost a relief when the miscarriage finally happened. During those four days I realized that doctors have so little to offer — they can't tell you what will happen, if the bleeding means that you are having a miscarriage, if staying off your feet really helps — they just don't know. I went to the hospital, had a blood test to check my hormone level, saw my doctor, and went home to bed.

The lab wasn't sure the test results would be ready the next day, a Friday: I might have to wait until Monday. It's strange how all my energy came to be focused on the results of that blood test, even though I knew that it wouldn't tell us very much. I knew that if the hormone level was low, it was fairly certain that the pregnancy wouldn't last. If it was high, then maybe I was not having a miscarriage after all. I continued to bleed; by Monday, I would be able to tell them, and the blood test would be irrelevant. Nevertheless, I called the lab every fifteen minutes.

I went to work Friday afternoon because it was my first day on a new job, and I felt it important to be there, even if only for a few hours. My husband picked me up at my car and drove me to the building my office was in so I wouldn't have to walk the two blocks. Although there was no reason to think that walking would hurt, we didn't want to take the chance. I called the lab every time I had a free moment between clients. By 5:00, they thought they'd have a result for me before the weekend. It turned out to be OK, a reasonably high HCG, which cheered me up a great deal. However, in the next few days my optimism proved to be ill founded.

I stayed in bed until Sunday. By that time, I'd had some pretty severe cramping and I began to wish for some resolution. The intensity of my feelings was getting to be too much for me; the only escape was sleep.

I had several hours of labor Sunday night. It stopped and started again at four or five on Monday morning. By seven or so, I had passed some tissue, which I could not bring myself to save in a jar, although I knew I should. My doctor had asked that I save any solid fragments so that he could make a diagnosis of why the pregnancy failed. But the thought of my would-be child in a container was too upsetting. When I felt something coming, I ran to the toilet, looked quickly, and flushed it down. I still believe it was the only thing I could have done.

So we went empty-handed to the hospital, my husband calling to cancel his day, and me calling to cancel mine before we walked out the door. I called one or two of my closest friends to tell them what was going on, then we left off our son with his sitter, as though it were a normal day.

In truth, by this time, I felt almost euphoric. The uncertainty was finally over. I'd go to the hospital, have a nice, antiseptic, sleepy cleanout, wait the required months and have another pregnancy. I felt that the preceding week had been the worst of my life. Now it was over and I could once again take control of what was happening to me.

The D and C went well, and I was able to leave the hospital that evening. I took the next day off from work to get myself back together: I needed to adjust to not being pregnant anymore. I took a long, glorious walk that day. It was one of the really crisp, sunny days of January with a brilliant blue sky, preceding the mush and gloom of February and March in Boston. I reveled in being able to move without worrying about whether I was bleeding or not —it didn't matter anymore. In fact, the more I bled, the more I felt cleansed of the whole mess. For the first time since I had become pregnant, I didn't feel anxious about moving the wrong way or too fast. I felt as though a weight had been lifted.

The euphoria, the sense of regained control over my body and my life, lasted for exactly one week. During that week I convinced everyone I spoke with that I was FINE. After a few days of this, they all began to believe that I was back to normal, and they all returned to business as usual in their dealings with me. And then — without warning or precipitant — I crashed. I cried. I felt I couldn't stand it. I started feeling enraged that this had happened to me: I was angry that other people were going through their days normally while I was feeling the most intense grief I had ever known. A child of mine, along with all of the dreams, hopes, and fantasies I had for him, had died.

In the week following the miscarriage I began to mourn. The world lost its interest for me; I went through the motions of living feeling like a self-conscious, mechanical doll. I was aware of every move I made and every word I spoke, yet I didn't feel like me. I got up, I somehow struggled through the decision of what clothes to put on. I didn't bother with makeup because I had no energy to put it on, and it didn't matter what I looked like. I went downstairs and through the usual ritual of eating breakfast, but it didn't matter what went into my mouth; I hardly tasted the food. I would walk outside and drive to work daydreaming, in a daze. Much of the time I felt as though I were wrapped in a gauze dressing like a caterpillar in a cocoon. Nothing seemed to mean very much to me: I felt like an observer watching myself and everyone else going about the business of living, while I wandered around in a semi-invisible state. I was also pre-occupied with time. I counted the days over and over in an endless litany. How much time since the miscarriage; how long before we could start trying again; what fraction of the wait was over — down to the hour. Over and over and over and over.

The only thing that could draw me out of my deadness was when I could talk about what had happened to me. All of a sudden I became three-dimensional and animated, a complete person, alive. Of course the problem was that not everybody wanted to hear in full and vivid detail about every nuance of my miscarriage and its aftermath. In fact, very few people wanted to hear about it at all.

I began to feel a little crazy about needing to talk about it so much, and I think I may have used some unsuspecting people as listeners and sounding boards because I was so self-absorbed that I wasn't always aware of what the needs of the other person were. I was able to work fairly well, but daring my nonworking hours I had a lot of trouble listening to other people's concerns. There were some people I couldn't speak to at all — most especially, pregnant friends. I could not stand to hear someone complain in any way, shape, or form about anything that had to do with being pregnant when I felt that if only I were pregnant, everything would be OK. Those friendships really suffered.

AUGUST 1979

Despite how horrible I felt during those months, I think few people noticed. I think that part of the intensity of the isolation I felt was that I could fool people so well. It was clear to me that most people wanted to believe that everything was fine. Everyone was only too willing to accept my superficial smile and work-as-usual schedule as evidence that things were back to normal.

I had never noticed before how there are a million things to remind one of pregnancy. A television commercial for Pampers would make me cry. A woman walking down the street in a loose dress would fill me with envy. As the days became longer and spring established itself, I could only think that I wasn't beginning to "show" the way I thought I would be when the buds and flower started to bloom. I felt that every woman on the street could have some-

thing that I couldn't, something that I craved more intensely than I've ever desired anything in my life.

In addition, I was feeling exhausted. Everything seemed an incredible effort, from getting out of bed to washing my hair to dealing with my three-year-old son to picking up the telephone.

There was also less emotional energy than usual available for my child and my husband, because so much was consumed by my preoccupation with pregnancy. Although intellectually I knew that this was normal for someone as depressed as I, it nevertheless made me feel guilty.

My husband was as understanding as he could be, but he didn't comprehend what this had done to my whole sense of myself. He didn't understand why I wasn't consoled by the thought that I could have another pregnancy, and by already having one child. I worried about how little I had to give to our son. I felt at once overcome with our good fortune to have him and yet strangely angry with him and his demands.

It was a difficult time for my husband and me. I think that no matter how hard a woman tries to explain what it feels like to have her whole sense of herself as a creative being shaken, it is difficult if not impossible for a man to comprehend her experience on anything but an intellectual level. I'm sure that neither of us was prepared for how intensely upset I felt. After months of my moping and lack of interest, my husband finally confronted me with his feeling that by this time I should be able to have more perspective. I, of course, felt enraged by his insensitivity and resentful toward him for having escaped the full burden of the loss. I also felt confirmed in my sense of estrangement from him. In my heart of hearts, I began to wonder if the fault didn't lie with his sperm, rather than with my egg. Since that time I have learned that he suspected that the reverse was true. It seems that neither of us understood how deeply the loss had affected us individually and as a couple, and thus were unprepared for the many strong, and often irrational, feelings that emerged.

The very hardest single experience I had to face in the months after my miscarriage was a baby shower. The woman who invited me let me know sensitively that she would understand if I chose not to come, but that she wanted to give me the option of attending if I wanted to. Needless to say, it was a painful decision, and I was obsessed over what I should do until the hour at which I knew I'd have to leave if I were going to get there in time. I finally decided to go, in part because the guest of honor had herself been through a miscarriage, and she had talked endlessly with me about the depression and self-doubt that had followed for her, and in part because it felt so self-indulgent and dramatic not to go that I knew it could only further lower my self-esteem if I gave in to the urge to bury myself for the duration. It was a sad evening for me. I had to try hard not to let my ever-present sadness show at such a joyous gathering. Yet how could there be anything else on my mind as I stared at my friend's ripe, round, beautiful body, and the proud bellies of several other of the guests as well. I felt shrunken, devalued and useless, being unable to carry out this most wondrous of tasks.

I waited the required three months before putting away my diaphragm. Those first three periods were each welcomed with celebration, because it meant one less month to delay. Especially the first signaled to me that things were on their way back to normal, my body was cycling, and we hoped it would be a short time before we'd be trying to conceive again. Nevertheless, not being able to try when we wanted a baby so badly was extremely hard to tolerate. Time passed very slowly because I knew there was nothing to hope for.

We didn't conceive in the first cycle when we tried, and that was a big disappointment. It felt as though all the waiting and anticipation of the past four months built up to a climax in the days before my period was due. I even felt convinced that I was having symptoms of pregnancy. My mind played every trick: there was a little fullness to my breasts, a little nausea, a little extra tiredness. And then the blood came. I tried to pretend to myself that it wasn't really my period, that it was the kind of bleeding you can have and still be pregnant. When I could no longer pretend to myself that it wasn't really my period, I cried long and hard for the baby I had lost and the anguish I had felt, for the baby we hadn't started yet, and I cried for myself. It all came back in a giant, overwhelming rush — and I cried for it all, in frustration and helplessness, all over again.

POSTSCRIPT

JUNE 1980

It has been fifteen months since my miscarriage. Much of the writing was done during the time of my own bleak mourning, as an attempt to gain control of my feelings by putting them on paper, hoping to console myself as well as anyone who might someday read this. I am especially happy to be writing now that we have a second healthy son. I feel that I love him all the more for having gone through such hell before he came to us.

During the time I was pregnant with him, and particularly during the first trimester, I was unable to either look at or continue this account. In fact, I was almost too anxious to tell anyone that I was pregnant or to acknowledge to myself that this pregnancy felt totally different to me, and much more "right." I was quite sure that I could not bear to go through another miscarriage.

Now that it is behind me, I am happy to report that one does get over the anguish and the pain — if not completely, then enough to have the intensity of it dulled by the passage of time, and, it is to be hoped, by the birth of a child.

3. Stillbirth — The Death of a Child

Despite the best efforts of the medical profession, little is known about what causes stillbirth. More often than not, the pregnancy is normal and uneventful until, suddenly, fetal movement ceases for longer than twenty-four hours, bleeding occurs, or labor starts.

The diagnosis is stillbirth, defined as the death of the fetus between the twentieth week of pregnancy and birth. Death may be detected while the fetus is still in the uterus, or possibly not until labor is underway, or until the baby is delivered. In the United States one stillbirth occurs for every eighty live births.

WARNING SIGNS

Women whose stillbirth is detected before labor begins frequently have a warning sign such as vaginal bleeding or cessation of fetal movement for longer than twenty-four hours. They may experience pain in the pelvis, lower abdomen, or back. Or one or more of the symptoms of toxemia may be present: rapid, unexplained weight gain; swelling of the fingers, ankles, and eyelids; headache; or visual difficulties. At times, premature labor is the first danger signal.

Your doctor is the best judge of whether your symptoms are severe enough to indicate a problem. He or she will want to know as many details as possible, so that he or she can make an accurate assessment.

Absence of Fetal Movement

Babies differ greatly in how active they are. It is normal for women not to feel the baby kick for hours at a time. However, if the baby has not moved at all for twenty-four hours, it is cause for concern and your physician should be informed.

Bleeding

At any time during pregnancy, bleeding is a sign there may be trouble, yet the majority of women who bleed during pregnancy go on to carry the baby to term. If bleeding occurs, you should consult your doctor.

Pain

Persistent or severe pelvic pain such as cramping, heaviness, sharp stabbing, or contractions are other signs of trouble. Your doctor will want to know what type of pain you are having, how intense it is, and whether the pain is intermittent or constant.

Fetal Heartbeat

A significant sign of fetal life is a heartbeat, which can usually be detected as early as the middle of the fifth month of pregnancy. As part of routine prenatal care, physicians listen for a fetal heartbeat. If the physician cannot find a heartbeat and suspects a stillbirth, he or she may order an ultrasound examination. This diagnostic aid allows him to visualize the fetus directly and to determine if a heartbeat is present. If a heartbeat still cannot be detected, stillbirth is then diagnosed.

COPING WITH THE FIRST SIGNS OF TROUBLE

Most women, when they see that first drop of blood, become concerned about pain, or realize that the baby has not moved for "too long," experience a "sinking feeling in the pit of the stomach." While they may fear that something is wrong, they may not want to face the possibility that they might lose the baby. It is common to feel emotionally frozen and to deny that there may be a problem — even to the extent of telling oneself that one was just imagining things. A woman probably considers phoning her doctor, but she may feel that she would be needlessly interrupting him, that she is being an "hysterical woman."

These are common reactions, but this is not the time for stoicism. She should tell her physician immediately if she is experiencing any of the warning signs. If the doctor cannot be reached, or is not responsive to the patient's concerns, it is wise to visit the emergency room of a good nearby hospital. It is better to err on the side of being too concerned.

The Bad News

If you have experienced symptoms and fear bad news, ask your husband or a friend or relative to accompany you to the doctor's office or the hospital. Your suspicions may be confirmed if the physician fails to detect a fetal heartbeat, or if he discovers that the uterus has failed to grow or has decreased in size, and if ultrasound examination fails to demonstrate the embryonic sac or the fetal heartbeat. If stillbirth is diagnosed, prepare yourself by asking your physician to describe what will happen, step by step. Your ability to cope with the physical and medical aspects of stillbirth will be improved if you are well informed. Your husband or a friend should hear this information as well, since it is possible that you may be feeling too upset to comprehend or remember very much.

SPONTANEOUS OR INDUCED LABOR

When stillbirth occurs prior to labor, the mother usually goes into labor spontaneously and delivers within about two weeks. However, this is not always the case. Sometimes labor may not begin for a month or more after stillbirth has occurred.

Because a woman who carries a dead fetus for more than four weeks has a 25 percent chance of developing a severe blood clotting disorder, known as intravascular coagulation, the pregnancy is always terminated well before the fourth week after intrauterine death.

Until recently, when stillbirth occurred prior to delivery, there was no alternative but to carry the pregnancy until labor began spontaneously, because there was no safe way to induce labor and cesarean section carried significant risks. Now, labor may be safely induced at any time after stillbirth is discovered using one of the prostaglandins.

Carrying a stillborn baby until labor begins is an emotionally distressing experience that most women prefer to avoid. For this reason most women choose to have labor induced as soon as possible. However, such is not the case for everyone. Some women prefer to carry the pregnancy in the hope that labor will begin spontaneously before two or three weeks have passed. This alternative is chosen by some women who prefer that labor and delivery be as natural as possible, and by others who wish to be with their child as long as they can. The final choice should be left to the individual, unless there are overriding medical considerations.

In discussing her decision to have labor induced, Catherine said: "I previously had a miscarriage in which I spotted for three weeks before it ended. The waiting was terrible — they were days lost out of my life. Every day I lay on the couch and hoped and waited and sometimes cried. During my second pregnancy, when my doctor diagnosed stillbirth, I asked for labor to be induced as fast as possible, and I entered the hospital the next morning."

Another woman, Janet, chose to await spontaneous labor, explaining, "Rationally, I knew my baby had died (at eight and a half months), but I couldn't yet choose to start labor. My husband and I wanted time to get over the shock, if possible, before labor and delivery. As it turned out, we had six days before labor started. I cried and Roy and I comforted each other during those days. In the hospital, he stayed with me and helped me through labor and delivery, using the techniques we learned in a natural childbirth class. All along, we had wanted everything to be natural, and we stuck to that even though we knew the baby was dead."

LABOR AND DELIVERY

Because labor and delivery are events of great magnitude, you may have found yourself preoccupied by the physical aspects of what was happening to you. The considerable pain of labor and delivery may have absorbed you and led you to suppress your feelings about your baby's death until after delivery. On the other hand, you may have been constantly feeling emotional pain over your loss and the irony of going through labor and delivery. Many women are anxious about their lack of knowledge and preparation for labor and delivery, fear surgery in the case of a cesarean section, and are apprehensive about hospitalization.

Some women have felt that it was preferable to be awake and aware during the delivery of a stillbirth because it helped them to experience the reality of what happened. Others requested general anesthesia, though it is not medically feasible for everyone.

Women who have experienced warning symptoms or who have received the diagnosis of stillbirth before delivery are naturally better prepared for the bad news. Others who have enjoyed normal, uncomplicated pregnancies are stunned to find out during labor or delivery that the baby is dead. This is the most difficult time to learn about a baby's death. Their expectations were high then and they were happily anticipating seeing their baby soon. Learning of the baby's death at this time is a tremendous blow; when compounded by the pain of the birth, the combined impact may be overwhelming. In addition, the labor and delivery staff are in all likelihood unprepared for what happened, and therefore shocked, upset, and unable to offer the support the mother so badly needs.

VIEWING THE BABY

Shortly after delivery, the patients are confronted with deciding whether to see the stillborn baby. Each couple must decide for themselves whether or not they choose to see or hold their dead infant. The most effective role of the staff is to avoid making the decision for the parents, but to support them in whatever decision they reach. Seeing the baby should not be imposed on them, but offered, as people have different feelings and these feelings should be respected.

Sarah and John decided to see their baby. Sarah described the experience: "My husband said it was a girl and she was really beautiful. He told me he thought I should see her and I said OK. I knew this was my only chance and I might be sorry later if I didn't. The nurse brought the baby in, all wrapped up in a blanket. We both looked at her and touched her. She looked perfect, which was nice. It was a kind of a closure. We made a baby and she died."

Hospital practice and policy regarding seeing a baby that is dead varies tremendously. Many times the attitude of the individual doctor or nurse on duty determines how the situation is handled. Couples may either be encouraged to see the baby or discouraged from seeing it. In some instances, the matter is not brought up at all and must be initiated by the parents themselves. A couple has a right to see and hold their baby if they want to and should make the request if the opportunity is not offered. Sometimes, deterioration of the infant's skin has begun if the baby has been dead in the uterus for a few days; in other cases, the fetus may have a visible abnormality. Even in such instances, parents should be allowed to see the baby if they wish to. The staff should prepare them for what they will see. For many people, imagining the baby's appearance is very much worse than seeing and knowing.

One woman said: "Even though the baby was very tiny, I would have liked to have seen it at some point. I grieved so long for a baby with no face. I think seeing it would've helped me deal with the death better and I would've gotten over it faster. I used to stop and look at kids on the street and in stores and wonder if my child would've looked like that. People should have the option of seeing a dead baby. I would've liked to have seen it. I *still* would like to see it if I could."

For others, viewing the baby helps in the grief process. "It is much easier, I think, to grieve for a son, a person, seen, felt, touched, as opposed to not knowing. (And what a monstrous image we could have conjured up!) Seeing him erased my doubts of his existence or general condition. Seeing him helped to focus our grief — on someone who was."

Similarly, a young mother said: "I saw him. It was helpful. I wish I had a picture. He looked so peaceful, as if he was asleep, unlike the way I imagined him in his struggle with death."

However, some people choose not to view the baby and later feel it has been the right decision. Alice, a secretary, said: "We didn't want to see the baby. We felt it would be too hard on us, that it would imprint the death too strongly in our minds. My mother viewed the baby for us. She said she was beautiful and normal-looking. Somehow, her word was enough and a comfort to me."

In the last few years several hospitals have begun the practice of taking a photograph of all stillborn babies. The photograph is given to the parents if they want it. If the parents do not want it, the picture is kept, in case they wish to have it at some future time.

FUNERAL ARRANGEMENTS

Parents need to make decisions regarding religious ceremonies and arrangements for the stillborn baby's body. Many do not want the additional stress of any type of ceremony and ask the hospital to take care of all the arrangements. For others, the various steps in making arrangements — deciding whether to have a ceremony, naming the baby, the possibility of burial with a headstone, and other considerations — help in facing the reality of their loss. To them, the gathering of supportive and sympathetic family members and friends at religious rites are considered beneficial in dealing with their grief. The ceremony may also underscore the reality of their loss and the finality of it, helping them to face their loss and to grieve.

Because the death of your stillborn may be the first death you have encountered in your family, you may be unaware of religious practices. Generally, Protestant and Catholic clergymen follow the desires of the parents regarding ceremonies for a stillborn baby, while the Jewish faith does not recognize a baby until after it is one month old, so no formal ceremony is available.

A funeral service for a stillborn child is rare. In some Protestant denominations, a memorial service is held, if desired, within several weeks or a month. Family and friends gather for prayers, hymns, and meditation, often centering on the joy of resurrection, in a spiritually uplifting service.

Some couples prefer only a simple graveside service where the body or ashes are interred.

A Catholic priest said he is sometimes called to the hospital following a stillbirth, where he prays with and comforts the parents. Most often, he is contacted by the husband or wife several weeks after delivery. "They will request a special mass to be attended by family and friends. It is part of their grieving process." Also possible is a graveside service. Here again, the emphasis is on what the parents want and need.

Some couples derive great comfort from a religious service. For others it is an ordeal to be suffered through. The decision to have a service or to avoid such things should be yours alone and your wishes should be respected.

THE HOSPITAL STAY

The hospital stay, especially after delivery, is often traumatic. You probably haven't forgotten one detail of your experience and wish you had done some things differently.

You may have been in the hospital for the first time in your life and found hospital routines to be unfamiliar, upsetting, and intimidating. Possibly you preferred to do what you were told rather than to stress your personal preferences. Like most, you probably felt extremely vulnerable and had difficulty in arranging to have your needs met.

It is our experience that when women take control, their hospital stay tends to be a less painful one. Most people feel much less frightened if they know what to expect. It is always reasonable to request information about what has happened to you and about what is expected to happen next.

Most women find that having their husband, or a close friend or relative, with them during labor and delivery is helpful. It is routine practice in some hospitals to permit the husband to be with his wife during labor and delivery, or in the case of surgery, with her during premedication and recovery. In other hospitals, special permission may be required.

It is probably a good idea for *any* pregnant woman to consider whether, if the pregnancy should be lost, she would prefer to be separated from other obstetric patients during labor and recovery. If you would prefer your postpartum stay to be in the gynecology or surgical area, tell your doctor and hospital personnel and *insist* on getting what you want. Be prepared to be told that your request is "against hospital regulations" or that you are an "impossible patient." Despite the temptation to back down and withdraw your request, do not do so. Several days of seeing babies and happy parents can be far more unsettling than an irritated nurse or administrator.

Many women who recovered in the maternity ward found it extremely painful. "I was placed in a combination maternity-gynecology floor," said Karen. "This was a very emotionally upsetting experience. It might sound like I was trying to hide from the real world, but I found it very difficult to be surrounded by what I couldn't have. It was almost as if someone was rubbing it in my face. I was on a happy floor and I was far from being happy. I learned very quickly to stay in my room with the door shut when the nursery cribs were being rolled past my door. In fact, I didn't like walking in the hall at all."

Seeing happy parents with their babies can be traumatic, some women feel. Being in a ward with happy mothers caused many women to hide their feelings lest they spoil the happiness of others.

"I went home as soon as possible," one woman said. "There was a woman on the other side of the curtain with her family admiring their healthy baby. It tore me apart not to have mine."

Several women commented that they would have coped better if they had been in private rooms. "I wish I'd had a private room. I was unable to cry, so I held back my emotional feelings. I didn't want to disturb my roommate. I couldn't tell my husband how I felt, because my roommate was always there."

On the other hand, some women find that isolation in a private room adds to their feelings of failure, guilt, and misery. They are less lonely sharing a room with one or more women and think it is an advantage to be with others. "I was glad to have an understanding woman in the next bed. She was recovering from surgery. She listened to me and encouraged me to talk about how bad I felt. It was especially good to have her there late in the evening after my husband left."

Many couples who have experienced a stillbirth want to remain together throughout the hospital stay. If you want your husband to stay with you, you or he should negotiate this with the floor personnel. If you have a private room, the staff may be willing to put a cot for him in your room. There will likely be times when you feel you want to be by yourself or alone with your spouse and you should communicate this. Hospital personnel should respect your wish for privacy. Also, let them know whether you want visitors. Many women want unrestricted visiting of friends and relatives, and this should be arranged if you desire it.

It is reasonable to request that your doctor inform all hospital personnel on your floor about your situation so that you are dealt with appropriately. A thirty-year-old computer programmer related her experience after a stillbirth: "Nurses came in and asked me several times if I had a name for my baby yet. I couldn't believe they didn't read my chart to know what happened to me. I was still in shock and I couldn't believe I was in a maternity ward. I did OK in the hospital, but kind of mentally collapsed when I got home — the whole experience was a total nightmare."

The lack of communication with your doctor, nurses, and other hospital staff members can be troubling. "I feel that my medical needs were met; however, there was no support for my emotional needs," one young woman said. "The doctor and the hospital personnel seemed not to know what to say, so they just acted very 'professionally' towards me. If the staff had simply acknowledged the fact that I did feel emotional pain, or even at least acknowledged that I felt something it could have helped."

The main criticism that couples who have experienced a fetal loss have about the care they received while in the hospital is that nursing and medical personnel were not sufficiently available to them. Feeling that the staff avoided them, rather than offering sympathy and emotional support, was common. Women report that one distressing aspect of hospitalization is the isolation they feel. The lack of attention to the tragedy that has hit them is another. Repeatedly, women told us of the need to talk to someone, to have their feelings of intense sadness validated and to seek acceptance. Avoidance by the hospital staff only fostered feelings of unworthiness and guilt.

"I had a terrible hospital experience," the mother of a stillborn baby said. "Few, if any, offered support. Some were not aware of the experience and no one talked about the death. I wanted to talk, but no one gave me the opportunity or freedom to."

Generally, couples were relieved and grateful when medical personnel responded with sympathy and concern. Many women praised the invaluable support that they received from their doctors and nurses. They were appreciative when staff members listened to them talk about their feelings or acknowledged that they had had a difficult experience. Most felt that when they were treated sympathetically and allowed to express their grief openly, they tended to feel better. As Donna said: "I was in a private room and felt isolated. Nurses and staff members came in to talk to me — to relate similar experiences. This helped me cope, knowing I wasn't alone.

"And my doctor talked to me several times in the hospital. He said that he realized what this pregnancy meant to us. Although he was reassuring about future pregnancy, he acknowledged the grief I felt for this one. He even said that this was a very sad time and that I should feel free to cry. For some reason, I needed his permission to cry and I will always be thankful for this man's understanding and kindness."

Nurses, in particular, may be open to offer emotional support, but are often reluctant to initiate discussion for fear of invading your privacy. It may be up to you to approach them.

THE POSTPARTUM PERIOD

The postpartum period is the time between delivery and the return of the pelvic structures to their nonpregnant state. Generally, this takes about six weeks. For women who have had normal pregnancies, it is a difficult time of adjustment. For women who have lost their babies, the period is exceptionally stressful, both physically and emotionally.

During her postpartum hospital stay of one to three days, a bereaved woman is often still in shock and only beginning to face the depth of her feelings of loss. In addition to the emotional distress that she feels at this time, she will probably also experience some physical discomfort. This physical discomfort may be hard for her to bear because her ability to cope with stress is impaired. In addition, it may be a reminder that her body has been preparing for motherhood and this preparation has been for nought.

Physical Concerns

LOCHIA The first physical process a woman is likely to experience is vaginal discharge (lochia) from the site of placental attachment to the uterus. This usually begins during delivery and continues for up to a month afterward. At first, the lochia will be red. Over a few weeks, it will change to brown and then to a yellow-white discharge.

AFTERPAINS Immediately after delivery the uterine muscles contract. This blocks exposed uterine blood vessels, keeping bleeding to a minimum. When this happens, many women will experience abdominal cramps much like menstrual cramps or labor pains. These cramps, or afterpains, are usually most intense right after delivery has occurred. Thereafter, they decrease in intensity and frequency. Some women have afterpains for a day or two following delivery.

EPISIOTOMY Like many women, you may find stitches and the healing incision from the episiotomy uncomfortable to the point of being unable to sit in a hard chair or car seat for up to three weeks. Sitting on a pillow or inflatable "doughnut" is helpful, as well as taking a warm tub or sitz bath in about four inches of water but without soap or bubble bath. Gently patting the perineal area with a soft, clean cloth may also help. It is preferable to take a shower, rather than a bath, during the first three weeks postpartum to avoid the possibility of infection.

MILK IN BREASTS Many women who have had a second-trimester miscarriage or a stillbirth find that on the second to fourth day after delivery their breasts become engorged with milk. Since one's body has no way of knowing that the fetus has died, it automatically prepares for breast feeding. Engorgement may cause some physical discomfort, but normally the actual physical pain is less troublesome than the emotional pain that may accompany it. Barbara described finding that her breasts were full of milk as "nature's cruel joke." Like many women, she was both surprised and horrified to find that her body was preparing to feed a child that would never be.

Sarah commented, "My breasts were bothering me, and when I would think of them being full of milk, sometimes tears would fill my eyes and sometimes I would feel angry. It seemed so unfair that I had all this milk, but no baby to feed it to. Something else that I found disturbing was that I had spent several months preparing my nipples and breasts for feeding, attended classes, expecting to nurse. Now in the hospital I was trying to stop the milk."

We would like to offer several suggestions for dealing with breast engorgement. First, you should not squeeze your breasts, since this will result in further production of milk. To relieve discomfort, wear a tight bra to bind the breasts, apply ice packs or hot wet compresses, or take an aspirin or other mild pain-relief tablet. The milk will soon dry up of its own accord.

Postpartum Blues

Most women are noticeably affected by the rapid and dramatic decrease in reproductive hormone levels which occurs at the time of delivery. Many experience physiological depression, irritability, and mood swings caused by hormone withdrawal; these feelings are commonly known as "milk blues." Usually the postpartum depression is relatively mild; however, in a woman who has had a stillbirth, this depression can compound an already present grief reaction.

A happy mother with a healthy baby may suddenly find herself in tears because her emotional threshold is unusually low. However, chances are this is a time-limited problem and in a matter of days, or at most a few weeks, she will feel better. In contrast, the mother of a stillborn baby might find the combination of profound grief and physiological depression to be distressing and overwhelming. Weeks may pass with no decrease in the intensity of her emotions. She may feel depressed, out of control, irritable, and unable to cope.

Other Concerns

Generally, during the postpartum period women tend to feel fatigued and depressed. That is why it is important to get lots of rest. Seek help with whatever household or other tasks seem too much for you. And of course, you should recuperate fully before returning to your job and a demanding schedule.

Sexual relations can be resumed three weeks after delivery if the stitches have healed, the vagina feels all right, and all bleeding and discharge have stopped.

Normally, your first menstrual period will start in about a month to two months after delivery.

Any unusual signs or symptoms should be reported to your doctor. These include fever, with or without chills; heavy vaginal bleeding; unusual breast or abdominal pain; and painful urination.

LOSING WEIGHT Following stillbirth a number of women report difficulty coping with the weight gain of pregnancy and with still "looking pregnant," because the increased weight and change in body contours were associated with the baby inside them. Some women become obsessed with losing weight and getting back to their normal size. They join exercise classes and go on strict diets in an effort to erase at least the physical signs of the failed pregnancy. They may gain some satisfaction in the ability to control this one facet of their lives, feeling that everything else is out of their hands. Other women may lack interest in their weight and appearance. Because they feel depressed, they may use food as a source of satisfaction. Whatever your reaction, your diet and exercise plan should be checked out with your doctor and any rapid loss or gain of weight avoided.

CAUSES OF STILLBIRTH

Once a stillborn baby is delivered, parents and medical staff members become concerned with what caused the death. Among the known causes of stillbirth are chromosomal abnormalities, umbilical cord accidents, placental problems, and toxemia. However, it is not uncommon that no cause is found, even after an examination of fetal and placental tissues and an autopsy of the infant.

Stillbirth occurs at the rate of 12.6 for every 1,000 live births (Indiana Vital Statistics, 1972). The following chart shows the number for each major cause of stillbirth per 1,000 live births.

Umbilical cord accidents and placental problems	4.5
Congenital malformations	1.0
Unknown causes	2.5
Fetal disease	2.1
Maternal obstetric complications	1.7
Maternal medical problems	0.6

Cord Accidents

Umbilical cord accidents pose a threat to a fetus because they may cause the oxygen supply through the cord to be cut off. Sometimes the cord develops a knot or coils around the fetus's neck or body so tightly that oxygen is shut off or interrupted, resulting in either fetal death or damage. Most cord accidents occur during labor and delivery, although they can cause intrauterine death prior to labor. They are unlikely to happen to the same mother more than once.

Placental Disorders

Severe placental problems can cause fetal death as well. In placenta previa, the placenta is implanted low in the uterus instead of in its normal location high on the anterior or posterior (front or back) wall of the uterus. Evidence of placenta previa is usually painless vaginal bleeding in the last trimester of pregnancy. The blood is bright red and the flow may range from light to heavy. The baby is unaffected unless the mother's blood loss is severe and results in a decrease in the oxygen supply to the fetus.

Another placental problem is premature separation of the placenta from its site of implantation in the uterus. Separation is considered premature if it occurs anytime before delivery. It is most common in the third trimester, but can happen at any time after twenty weeks. The seriousness depends on whether the separation is partial or complete. Placental separations range from very partial ones, which may be largely asymptomatic and have no evident effect on the fetus, to severe separations, which lead to excruciating uterine pain, hemorrhage, and fetal death.

Genetic Factors

Genetic studies should be carried out to determine whether either parent or the fetus carries a chromosomal abnormality. If this is found, genetic counseling is advised before another pregnancy is conceived.

Toxemia

Severe toxemia accounts for 3 deaths per 100,000 live births and can lead to maternal death as well. There is no known cause of toxemia, which is characterized by the development of high blood pressure, retention of fluid in the body, and protein in the urine.

Symptoms include sudden and excessive weight gain, swelling of the fingers and ankles and puffiness of the eyelids; headache; and disturbances in vision. Toxemia can be mild and produce no lasting difficulties for either the mother or her baby. When it is diagnosed in its early stages and medical advice is followed, the more severe consequences of the disorder can be prevented.

Other Factors
There are many other factors that may cause stillbirth, including maternal illness, either infectious or systemic (such as diabetes); complications of labor or delivery; Rh factor incompatibility (almost always preventable); and severe nutritional deficiency.

One Woman's Story

One year later. Somehow it seems like only yesterday. The weather is much the same — naturally — though it is hard to recall much about the weather then. Only that during my labor (in August) I somehow convinced the nurse to turn on the heat and bring blankets. And the way it rained, soft and cool and so green, the day they buried the baby.

I had a very easy pregnancy — only the most minor complications — had no morning sickness — felt and looked remarkably healthy. Starting from the first visit to the doctor, at ten weeks, there was not the slightest hint of any difficulty. My chart consistently showed "0" risk. There were of course the jokes and rebukes about my weight gain, which was considerable. Not to say those visits were easy — the doctors always seemed concerned and helpful — but there was always the nagging thought "Does he remember me, or know my name without referring to my chart?" Perhaps it was sheer unreasoned anxiety, simply a case of being overwhelmed by one's emotions. Later, my hand would shake at the prospect of telephoning his office.

On the last scheduled doctor's visit before my due date I was full of eager anticipation. The nursery was set and I was looking forward to taking my leave from the office and having a few days at home for final preparations (I fully expected to deliver late). It was a summer day like many others. As was our usual routine, it was a late morning appointment, to be followed by lunch with my grandparents. Joseph dropped me off and left to do his usual errands.

My doctor's partner was on duty, and I went into his examining room, where the baby's heartbeat would be broadcast on a speaker near the table. Like always. First, the casual greetings. I told the doctor I hadn't noticed the baby moving for a couple of weeks. The doctor explained this was not uncommon at this stage, due to the larger size of the baby. He checked last Saturday's report — oh yes, Dr. B. had found movement.

Then the stethoscope was ready . . . no familiar sound . . . the phone rang, and the doctor casually left to reassure some other expectant mother. Soon he was back, and patiently resumed the search for the elusive heartbeat. Then he stopped.

I was confused, and asked naively, "Is this cause for concern?" He assured me it was. He manipulated my belly but got no response. He would not say anything; he only scheduled another appointment and remarked that he hoped I wouldn't still be waiting then.

Tears filled my eyes as I spoke with the nurse on the way out. I was confused, fearful, but not sure. Was the baby dead? If so, why hadn't the doctor told me?

Joseph was waiting, and I got into the car. In his usual fashion he would have had us at my grandparents' door in a half-minute, but I begged him to detour and find a place where we could sit and talk. I needed time to compose myself and tell him. We were still not sure. But we agreed not to tell my grandparents. Once there, we said little, and I went to the bathroom to cry as often as I could, and put on my best effort so as not to alarm them.

We left as soon as we could. I told Joseph there are times when only one's mother will do. We went to my parents' house, and Joseph told my father as I cried in the bathroom. My mother was at the town common at one of the local festivities, Autumn Fair.

We set out to find her. Searching through the crowd, my eyes found her in a lawn chair in a shady spot. I explained what had happened, and she, too, was concerned. A neighbor whose wife was due about the same time came by with a bright smile and cheery remarks. She shooed him away. We hugged for a while, and when I felt strengthened, Joseph took me home.

It was then I decided that one point of our childbirth classes had been the helpfulness of the nurses. Rather than endure this uncertainty, I called the labor and delivery unit. By luck Mrs. L., the head nurse, answered. I didn't know her then, only that there was a calm, understanding, patient woman at the other end of the line. I explained what had happened at the doctor's office, and asked her opinion. She erased my uncertainty and let me down very gently. "Why didn't the doctor tell me?" I asked. "You know, we're human, too. . . ." She wondered why the doctor hadn't informed her. Quick to defend him, I explained that it had only been a few hours since my appointment. Anyway, she asked a few questions and reassured me that she would be expecting me. I didn't quite grasp the importance of that until later.

So I began to get used to the idea. Try as I might, I could no longer stimulate any movement from within. At last there was no hope, and I had to think of what to do, to plan.

Mother called. She had discussed my case with a nurse friend, and had gotten an answer of little hope, but maybe a slight chance. She, like me, was grasping at straws. Now it was my turn to gently explain how I had talked to the nurse in labor and delivery, and that I no longer doubted. She didn't give up, though. She had talked to both my doctor and his partner at length by noon the next day, pressing them for answers.

Somehow the rest of the day and evening passed. I was determined to stay in the house — no more public places and friendly faces and cheery remarks. They meant well, of course, but I couldn't bring myself to risk the confrontation.

Joseph was very good. He came to understand even more slowly than I, and somehow buried his personal torment in his concern for me. He was anxious to throw himself into some sort of activity, but he refused to leave me alone.

Sunday midday. I sat on the deck soaking up the sun and trying not to think.

By Sunday afternoon Joseph arranged to take me to my mother's house for a while, and he then got away for a little. I sat in a nice straight-back chair and faced the television. We didn't talk much. It had gotten down to waiting. . . .

Back home, after dinner, there were at last decisions to be made. I had planned to work this week. My due date was Friday, but I had felt good, and had wanted to have the time off after the baby came rather than before. Moreover, I expected to be late. So my car pool was expecting me. On Saturday the doctor had said I could still go to work, but now the thought was appalling. So I decided that now was the time to get ready: wash hair, shave, and be ready. This done, my efforts at procrastination were about exhausted, and by nine o'clock I finally called a fellow in the car pool. I sadly explained that I would not be in, and would call when ready to return, sooner than I had planned.

We went to bed around ten. Now I was really hoping the time would come soon, that I would be spared this horrible waiting much longer. The lifeless baby was by now a burden, a source of frustration, such as he had never been in nine months. In the past I had chided him gently if he kicked a lot — now I would have given anything to feel such a little discomfort. Now he was just a lump, like a sack of potatoes. I hoped my time would come soon.

Mercifully we slept soundly until I was awakened by a sharp pain at 12:45 A.M. I was greatly relieved and was sure this was it. Before I had wondered if I would recognize the onset of labor. I had felt the Braxton Hicks contractions a lot late in my pregnancy, and once thought that might be what labor was. The doctor had laughed at my concern — after all, every woman knows. It feels like a contraction — well, how was I to know what a contraction feels like? It was not like anything I had experienced in the past, but I didn't press him too much because, after all, he never felt one, either. My sister had described hers, and her description was concrete enough, and exactly fit what I felt now. The bloody "show" was simply confirmation of what I already knew.

I called Mother and arranged for her to call our offices in the morning. Joseph was very nervous, and tried to rush me. But I lingered, fretting over the contents of my suitcase, sadly lacking baby things, only what I needed, and didn't need, for myself. I was terribly thirsty. Joseph made glass after glass of iced tea. Finally I was ready, and we set out for the hospital. At that point the pains were sharp but very short, and came at irregular but short intervals.

It didn't take long to get to the hospital. It was very dark and the roads were empty. We went to the emergency entrance as instructed. A nice little old man put me in a wheelchair, and, unknowing, tried to console me as I cried all the way to the maternity ward. Joseph followed after he had taken care of some paperwork.

The nurse was very nice and tried to cheer me up. "You're going to have a baby!" As I undressed in a little bathroom, Joseph quietly told her the unhappy circumstances. She then calmly prepped me, and in a perfunctory way put the stethoscope on my belly — no sound — for just the shortest time. Then I wanted to get up and move around. She sent us both in our white gowns to the fathers' waiting room. This room faced the nursery. We looked through and paced the floor and talked with a father-to-be who asked about my progress and told how his wife was doing. We didn't tell him.

Soon, the nurse came back and escorted us away from that depressing situation. We had asked for a private room, and she took us there now. It was a lovely large room, with one semicircular wall, all windows, overlooking a grassy area with trees. I remember especially the flowered wallpaper, which I would try to use later as a focal point for concentration.

I got into bed, with ginger ale and lollipops close by. Joseph settled into a comfortable chair, and we dozed. When the pains came, I called him to my side, and he always came, to help me, and when they subsided we napped again. Over and over from about 2 A.M. to daylight.

I remember the strangeness of the pains. When I got a strong one, I can remember thinking, This is the most horrible feeling in the world, and wondered how many children would be born if men had to bear them. At the same time, as the pain subsided, the relief was great. And when the pain was gone, it was just about forgotten. Was it really so bad??

Several times I had to go to the bathroom. Joseph's voice outside the door, over and over, queried, "Are you all right?" It was reassuring.

By morning the pains were getting stronger and Joseph valiantly tried to time them. I paid little attention, but often asked, "How often is it now?" At seven the doctor on duty was the same who on Saturday had found no life inside me. He advanced no farther than the doorway. Mrs. L., who had checked me shortly before, came with him. He asked two questions. He asked about the progress of my labor, to which Mrs. L. answered something, and he asked me if "anything had changed." I said only "no" and felt miserable. The look on his face, as Joseph later described it, was the look of death, an expression we shall never forget. I expect he felt truly sad — but at the time I was kind of disappointed that he didn't show more concern for me, that he did not examine me or even step towards me in the room.

In another way I was a little glad to think that this was his final round, and that my regular doctor would be on duty when I delivered.

Mrs. L. came in again. My mother had called, and she spoke with her. Again I felt reassured, not alone.

On one visit, Mrs. L. took over Joseph's job and helped me through a contraction. I was amazed at how much help another person could be. The other nurses had been nice, but lacked her authority. Even Joseph, whom I never promised to "obey," was less effective in this role. The adaptation of deep breathing — she taught me to let my belly rise on the inhale, hold, and fall on exhale — was much better for me than anything we did in childbirth class. Or maybe it was just her.

By eight o'clock I told Joseph I was losing my concentration and to ring for the nurse. Mrs. L. had just left, but the contractions were much stronger. Now she stayed with me. Into heavy labor. She checked me, positioned me, and leaned over me very close as we breathed together. It was as if we were one person. Soon it was really happening. I told her, "I feel something coming," and she said, "Let it go." It was the bag of waters breaking. She competently cleaned up. Now I really couldn't control — just let my head back in a kind of loud noise, more like a great groan than a scream. She pushed my head back down. "Don't let it out — push." It was at that time, about 8:30, she got the table and we went down to the delivery room. She advised Joseph to stay behind since she didn't expect it to be much longer. I was going to be given gas, as we had requested.

But I fooled her. I was not so eager as other women, knowing the outcome. We were in the delivery room for an hour before they finally put me under.

For some reason I thought the anesthetist and the doctor would not arrive in time. Anyway, I was not doing my best to hurry things along. I tried to sleep. I tried breathing instead of pushing. Watching the clock on the wall, I hoped it would be over soon, that I would be asleep and unaware of the rest.

Mrs. L. kept working with me. She called the doctor and the anesthetist. After a while I could see my doctor outside the delivery room. I could see his capped head over the top of a partition in front of the door. So he would not be late after all.

Finally at about 9:30 they all converged on me and decided I was ready. I felt like so much hamburger lying on the table, but felt relieved that the time had come and that these people would take care of me. I was just starting to fade out when I could feel a cool mist sprayed on my bottom — just a little bit of panic — I moved to show them I was still conscious, and someone said, "Wait a minute" — then I remember no more.

Awake and shaking, I saw only Mrs. L. still in the room. She was over near the wall in front of me doing something at a table. Joseph came in. He let out a scream, reeled, and punched the wall. She had shown him the baby. She ordered me to keep my head down.

Earlier Mrs. L. had asked if we wanted to see the baby. We had said no, but she advised us it would be better. Now I realized how right she was.

Joseph moved over by me, tears still in his eyes, and Mrs. L. gently brought the baby to me to hold. Like any other couple, our first question was "What is it?" A boy. And then, "How big?" Six pounds.

He had only been dead two or three days, so he looked very good — beautiful, as if asleep — wrapped in a blanket. Mrs. L. said not to open the blanket, as some skin had begun to deteriorate, but that there was no apparent abnormality. I held him for several minutes. I saw that he had Joseph's dark hair, and a little bow mouth. I felt stunned. I didn't know what to say or do. There were no tears then, just a sort of confused exhaustion, of being overwhelmed by this sad event.

I know now what I should have done — I sorely regret not having kissed him. Such a little thing. It just didn't occur to me until later, when it was too late. We also should have given him a name. He was and is very real to us — our son — but we had not agreed on a name before, and once we learned his sad fate, we somehow couldn't bring ourselves back to the question of a name. He should have had a name. We will forever now refer to him as "the baby." "The baby's room" is the nursery, his room, though he never slept in it.

Basically, we were ill prepared to cope with death. We both had been sheltered from other deaths, and had not suffered the loss of anyone close. So this was by far the greatest loss of our lives, not even close to any other.

I lay there gazing at the baby and finally Mrs. L. took him away and prepared me to return to my room. I was sort of relieved (I admit with some guilt) because it was just so sad, and I felt so powerless, so frustrated and confused.

We went back to my room about 11 o'clock and soon a nurse brought me lunch. I was hungry in spite of everything and ate most of it. Right away they wanted to know the name of the undertaker. This was another thing we had blocked from our minds and so were now shaken and had no answer. I got Joseph to call my mother for the name of the family friend, so that was taken care of. Joseph called his parents. We had decided not to tell them until after, since they live far away and there seemed no point in upsetting them any earlier. I had told my parents and my sister, and my mother told my grandparents and the people at our offices.

That afternoon I slept. Joseph roamed the hospital and went home to change. I ate my supper, and then worried that Joseph hadn't eaten. My mother came to visit, and my sister and her husband, whom I asked to take Joseph down to the cafeteria. Somehow concern over other things relieved a little of the greater grief. We both responded to the visitors — it gave us a chance for conversation, made us feel loved, and generally kept us going.

Joseph was allowed to stay past regular visiting hours, until about 10, when I went to bed.

Tuesday morning early I was awakened by the sound of babies crying. I wondered if any of the mothers were telling their babies not to cry, I thought how wonderful it would have been if my baby could cry.

My doctor came by around 7 and we talked. He said there was no apparent *cause of the baby's death. He said I was fine and could go home soon — not today, as I suggested, but preferably tomorrow morning. I accepted his advice. I specifically asked him whether he thought Rh incompatibility had been a problem. I knew that my blood type was B negative, that the Red Cross had told me I also had an antibody, anti-D, but that the blood test at twelve weeks had not shown the antibody. Joseph's blood type is B positive.*

I had no other blood tests until after delivery. At delivery I was not given RhoGAM [a preparation of immune globulin which prevents the production of anti-Rh-positive antibodies in the mother's blood]; the doctor said now that I was already sensitized [if antibodies are already present RhoGAM is ineffective]. The doctor said that blood disease was not the cause of the baby's death, that had that been the case there would be evidence, but that may be a problem in future pregnancies. An autopsy would be done, but the doctor was not hopeful of finding an answer — "Many times they don't."

The issue of blood type incompatibility would continue to haunt us, probably because that was the only questionable item of my health. I had brought the Red Cross letter on my first visit to the doctor, and at that time he ordered the hospital test, and said I would be retested later near term. The hospital's test did not show the antibody, and when I asked the doctor about it he said one of the two was wrong, probably the Red Cross. When it got to be close to my due date, I had asked each of the doctors if I would be retested. Each said no. It appeared to us that they were relying solely on the hospital's test, which was proven wrong in the end. Now we were told it was not the cause of death, but still it is a source of nagging doubt, and a problem for the future as well.

Joseph spent most of Tuesday with me, except for the visit to the cemetery he arranged, with the undertaker and our friend Bob. They went to see different sites, to decide on one, and to order a monument. He decided on a family plot where my great-grandparents are buried. There was room enough, the location is a quiet corner, and it seemed nicer not to bury the baby alone. The stone was to have a cross, Baby Boy A., and the date. We felt that in two or three weeks, by the time the stone was laid, we would be ready to go there for a brief service. My sister's husband is a minister and we asked him to lead the prayers.

One of my friends called. From the fellows in my car pool, the news had worked its way around to my former work location. I asked her to come visit and she did that evening. My parents both came, so for another day we were glad to have visitors, and loads of flowers and cards. Some I got later at home, and they were very important to us. We got all kinds of cards — sympathy, get well, cheer up — and personal notes. The words hardly mattered. It was the idea that these people cared and took the time to try to express their sadness and concern for us. I have saved them to this day.

Joseph left late again Tuesday night. That was the only complaint of my hospital stay — that he had to go at all. I missed him each night and wished that he could have slept there with me. And he was unhappy going home alone.

The nurses were very good to us. Each was friendly and helpful on their periodic visits. Mrs. L. was my special nurse, and with about thirty years' experience and six children of her own, she really knew the situation. Besides taking me through my labor and giving us the baby, she also made my bed and watched me closely. She hugged me and cried with me. It was like being under total care — physical and mental. I left her some of my flowers and later sent some fruit as a token, albeit inadequate, of our appreciation for her extraordinary care. Come to think of it, she watched us both — as she wheeled me to the delivery room, she ordered another nurse to get Joseph a glass of orange juice with sugar, because he looked pale.

Wednesday morning. I awoke early to the sound of babies crying. Today was the day I could go home. It was also the day the baby would be buried. I looked out at the rain and the green grass and cried.

The doctor came by as I finished my breakfast. There was no further information, just instructions on postpartum care. The printed instructions were for women in happier circumstances, of course. One part began, "When the baby is ten days old . . ."

I called Joseph and asked him to hurry. Finally he arrived and we prepared to leave. I had been dreading this moment. It seemed so sad to walk out empty-handed, past the glass-walled nursery. I clutched Joseph's arm and whimpered softly all the way to the car.

Home again. My sister and her husband came to see us that afternoon. Visitors again helping us by.

Wednesday night my milk came in. Tossing around in bed, there was this wetness. It seemed such a cruel blow that Mother Nature should do this to me now. Fortunately it didn't last, since I had had a shot in the hospital and had followed the nurse's advice.

Joseph stayed home with me and didn't go back to work until the following Monday. We had some visitors; mostly we stayed home. I felt safe being home. I dreaded going out, fearing I would see someone I knew, or that anyone might ask about the baby. I still looked pregnant — and I still walked like a pregnant woman. My reflection in a storefront window was enough to reduce me to tears.

When Joseph went back to work I found that for the first time I was alone for significant periods. I began to really learn the meaning of words — like anguish. *In my mind's eye I saw Edvard Munch's painting titled, I think,* The Scream. *That describes it better than words, and I felt it. I was more vulnerable now, since Joseph had hidden from me such things as the invoice for the baby's monument. Now I opened the mail alone — to find the bill from the undertaker, to find more cards, to find the final bill for the baby's monument. While all of this was hard to bear — I would cry, tear my hair — it was also a kind of catharsis that I was only able to accomplish when alone. I have a tendency to try to spare others my grief—if anyone asked about me, I would always answer "Fine" or at least "OK." Chin up, good front, and all that. Some maybe felt I suffered less because it didn't show too much. In any case it is true that I felt almost apologetic if a friend started to cry or evidenced sadness on my behalf. So it was really in this time alone that I had to face what had happened, and overcome the great desire to hide forever.*

I would have six weeks' total leave, so by the end of two weeks I started to go daily to a health spa. Also on Fridays I went into town to lunch with my working friends (I would arrange to meet them at the restaurant, so as to avoid seeing any other people I knew). Once a week or so I lunched with my mother, who would pick up some sandwiches on the way. The days fairly flew by as I occupied considerable time on these simple activities.

A few times I was aware how little people understand about these things. One friend (mother of two) at lunch remarked how with all this spare time I must be getting all my fall cleaning done. I simply said no. Couldn't she see it was the farthest thing from my mind? The minister surprised me, too. He stopped in to see me at the hospital. He prayed for me and Joseph and we talked. I had to ask him point-blank to say a prayer for the baby. While I appreciated his concern for us, it is, after all, the baby's death we are mourning.

My faithful visits to the figure salon had little effect, although I did try. I was to learn much later that the weight loss I sought would come chiefly with time (one year) and little or no effort. Another of life's mysteries.

The Sunday three weeks from the baby's birth the stone had been set and we had our memorial service. My grandparents, parents, brother, sister, and our friend Bob (who was to have been the baby's godfather) came, and my sister's husband led us in prayer. I brought an arrangement of white flowers. It was simple and personal and I cried straight through. It was the first time I had been to the gravesite, though I have been often since.

One year later, we went again, Joseph and I, and placed yet another all-white arrangement at the baby's grave. And marveled at how it doesn't seem like a year has passed.

4. Ectopic Pregnancy — A Compound Loss

"I had no warning. In fact, I had no idea what was going on until the emergency room nurse said it was an ectopic — a pregnancy in my right fallopian tube. Only then did it fit together. It was amazing how the shocky state I was in made me actually feel good and the deeper in shock I went, the better I felt.

"I realized at that point that there was nothing I could do to help myself or my husband. I knew he was very worried. It wasn't until several days after the surgery, when I was told that my chances of another ectopic were one in ten, that I began to comprehend what had happened to me and to feel the loss. Knowing I only had one tube left hit me very hard. I felt like my body had failed me.

"I felt frustrated and defeated. My husband was very distraught. He, more than I, realized how close to death I was. He was not willing to risk my life again for that of a possible baby."

Ectopic pregnancy. Before you had one you probably never heard of it. While you were in the middle of it you were probably stunned. You may have recently found out or not even have known you were pregnant. Then, suddenly, you were being rushed into the operating room. You woke up and learned that you had lost a baby and a fallopian tube. That's a tremendous loss, especially all at once. You are bewildered. "Why me?" you ask. "It's just not fair."

In the aftermath, you discovered very little is commonly known about ectopic pregnancy; many people you tell about it have never heard of it.

WHAT IS AN ECTOPIC PREGNANCY?

An ectopic pregnancy occurs when the fertilized egg implants itself outside the uterine cavity. By far the most common ectopic location is the fallopian tube (oviduct). This occurs in 95 percent of cases. Less commonly, the fertilized egg may implant in the ovary, the abdomen, or the cervix. Because it is most common, we will deal primarily with tubal pregnancy. Tubal pregnancy occurs approximately once in every 100 pregnancies in the United States.

Fertilization of the egg by the sperm usually occurs in the outer third of the fallopian tube. In a normal pregnancy, the egg is moved along through the tube by wavelike contractions and by the motion of hairlike cells, called cilia, which line the tube. After a journey of about two and one-half days, the egg reaches the uterine cavity, where it implants itself. If the passage of the egg through the tube is obstructed in any way, then it is possible that the fertilized egg may implant in the tube instead of proceeding on to the uterus.

If the egg implants in the tube, it may establish a placenta and begin to grow just as if it were in the uterus. This initial growth of the embryo can trigger the placenta to produce the hormones of pregnancy. If this happens, the usual signs of pregnancy may be present: missed menstrual period, breast fullness and tenderness, and nausea. The hormones produced by the ectopically implanted placenta may also induce uterine growth and softening of the cervix, so that a physician may be unable to distinguish it from a normal uterine pregnancy.

As the embryo grows, the tube expands initially; however, since it is not capable of marked expansion, continued growth will cause it to rupture. The extent to which the pregnancy develops and the way it terminates depends, in part, on where in the tube the implantation has occurred. Tubal pregnancies terminate in a variety of ways. If the fertilized egg dies in the tube prior to implantation, or if it dies soon after implantation has occurred, the embryo may be reabsorbed (through the blood vessels) without damaging the tube or causing any symptoms. If the embryo dies but is not reabsorbed, mild chronic symptoms, most characteristically anemia, may occur. If ectopic pregnancy is diagnosed before the tube ruptures, the embryo can be surgically removed, saving the tube. Tubal rupture occurs when the growing embryo breaks through the tubal wall, or when the trophoblast, the primitive placenta, invades and erodes the blood vessels of the tube, causing hemorrhage. This usually occurs about two weeks after the missed menstrual period or four weeks after conception. Rupture of the fallopian tube is a medical emergency and requires immediate surgery.

RUPTURED TUBAL PREGNANCY — SIGNS AND SYMPTOMS

Diagnosis of an unruptured ectopic pregnancy is extremely difficult because the majority of patients do not develop clearcut signs and symptoms. When a pregnant woman develops severe abdominal pain in the first trimester, the possibility of ectopic pregnancy is usually considered. However, this possibility is sometimes overlooked when a woman who does not know she is pregnant experiences severe abdominal pain. If ectopic pregnancy is suspected, a very sensitive pregnancy blood test (measuring the beta subunit of HCG — human chorionic gonadotropin) is done. This test can detect the low level of hormones produced by the ectopic pregnancy. If the beta subunit test is positive, a sonogram (a picture made with ultrasound) will be done to see if the fetal sac is located in the uterus.

Most of the signs and symptoms of tubal pregnancy are caused by stretching, the ultimate rupture of the tubal wall, and hemorrhage into the tube or into the abdomen.

Pain
This is the most common symptom of a ruptured tubal pregnancy. Pain may be localized on one side or present over the entire abdomen. It may be cramping, stabbing, or tearing, intermittent or continuous. Commonly, the pain extends upward to the shoulder or neck. It may be the first symptom noted, or it may occur along with or after bleeding.

Missed Menstrual Period

Seventy-five percent of women with ectopic pregnancies report missing a menstrual period. One quarter of the patients report that they did not miss a menstrual period. The bleeding associated with a tubal pregnancy may be mistaken for a normal period.

Vaginal Spotting and Bleeding

Vaginal bleeding is usually scanty and dark brown, and it may be intermittent or continuous. Severe vaginal bleeding rarely occurs in ectopic pregnancies. Profuse vaginal bleeding is more characteristic of miscarriage than of ectopic pregnancy, yet it occurs in 5 percent of all such cases.

Fainting and Weakness

These symptoms occur in about one third of women with ruptured tubal pregnancies and are caused by severe pain and hemorrhage.

Pain during Intercourse

Pain during intercourse sometimes is experienced with an ectopic pregnancy. Pain may result when the distended tube is jarred or when internal bleeding has occurred.

WHAT AN EXAM SHOWS

During a pelvic examination, movement of the cervix may cause severe pain. In 50 percent of patients, a tender pelvic mass can be identified to the side of or behind the uterus.

If bleeding has been significant, either into the abdomen or vagina, a decrease in blood pressure, an increase in pulse rate, and a drop in body temperature may result.

DIAGNOSIS

Because of the danger of hemorrhage, it is important to know the warning signs and to report them promptly when they occur. Since the consequences of a ruptured ectopic pregnancy are serious, it is best to err on the side of safety and to check out all concerns with your obstetrician.

Some other conditions mimic some of the signs and symptoms of ectopic pregnancy: pelvic inflammatory disease, threatened or in-complete miscarriage, an ovarian cyst, and appendicitis. The physician will take a detailed history, perform a physical examination, and probably also order some tests to help him make a diagnosis. Following are some of the tests used.

Common Diagnostic Procedures

CULDOCENTESIS Insertion of a needle through the vagina into the space behind the uterus to determine whether there is blood in the abdominal cavity. The presence of blood would indicate that tubal rupture has occurred.

POSTERIOR COLPOTOMY A surgical incision made in the vaginal wall to investigate whether blood has accumulated in the space behind the uterus. If it has, this is a sign that the tube has ruptured and that internal bleeding has occurred.

CULDOSCOPY Visualization of the abdominal cavity by means of an instrument inserted through an incision in the vagina.

LAPAROSCOPY A procedure in which an optical instrument called a laparoscope is inserted through a small incision in the abdominal wall. This procedure permits the doctor to visualize directly the fallopian tubes and other pelvic organs.

ULTRASONOGRAPHY Use of high-frequency, short-wavelength sound-wave reflections to determine whether the uterus is enlarged, whether a fetus can be visualized in the uterus, and whether an ectopic fetal mass can be distinguished outside the uterus.

PREGNANCY TEST In recent years pregnancy tests have become of greater value in diagnosing ectopic pregnancies. With early gestation only small amounts of the pregnancy hormones are produced, so it is not uncommon for a woman with an ectopic pregnancy to have a negative routine pregnancy test. Recently, however, the test for the beta subunit of HGC, described just above, has been available to aid in the diagnosis of ectopic pregnancy. Because it is able to measure lower levels of pregnancy hormones than could be determined by ordinary pregnancy tests, an ectopic pregnancy can be ruled out if this test is negative.

Treatment

Surgery is required whenever ectopic pregnancy is diagnosed or strongly suspected, even if the tube has not ruptured. Salpingectomy (removal of the entire fallopian tube) is the surgical procedure most frequently performed. Conservative surgery — that is, an effort to repair or reconstruct the damaged tube — is performed when the woman wishes to attempt pregnancy in the future and her other tube is nonfunctioning or absent, while the damaged tube appears to be salvageable.

There is, unfortunately, an increased risk of having a recurrent ectopic pregnancy after conservative surgery because adhesions or scar tissue may form and obstruct the tube. Yet for the woman who is anxious to conceive a child, this procedure may offer the possibility that her fertility can be preserved.

THE HOSPITAL STAY

Women who suffer an ectopic pregnancy often experience a series of upsetting events. Those who don't even know that they are pregnant may be completely baffled. Some women experience mild to moderate pain for a week or longer before the ectopic pregnancy is diagnosed or the tube ruptures. For others, acute pain is the first sign of trouble. Whatever the duration or nature of the pain, the dramatic symptoms of ectopic pregnancy, including blood loss, pain, and shock, can be terrifying. As with many other women, it may have been your first serious medical ailment and likely your first brush with death.

Because the surgery was done under general anesthesia, you probably woke up, following surgery, in the recovery room, with an intravenous tube, feeling nauseated, groggy, disoriented, and in pain. You were probably heavily medicated — a period of grace. As the medication wore off, the reality struck you.

Shortly after you woke up, your husband or your doctor told you what had happened. Chances are the message you got was a minimized or understated version to avoid alarming you. Most doctors try to soften the blow at first. Your physician may have told you of the damage to your fallopian tube and what measures he had taken, but he may have held off from discussing the implications for future pregnancies.

Several women said that their initial reaction was to feel relief that they had survived after coming so close to death. Only later did they begin to recognize what they had lost.

Following surgery, you are usually hospitalized for from four to six days. Some women told us that being placed in the obstetrics area was particularly difficult. They felt that facing new mothers and babies was extremely traumatic as they realized the loss of their own child and possibly their fertility as well.

"It was worse for me emotionally than physically," Marge said. "I was on the obstetrics floor after my ectopic for five days, surrounded by happy mothers and fathers and their babies. I was particularly sensitive to seeing them because I had lost a baby and a tube. I was very distressed I might not ever have a baby as we had hoped and planned. When I got home, I could let go of my emotions, and I felt much better."

Some women felt that they were treated merely as surgical patients; their emotional needs were not met. Jane talks about her six-day hospital stay: "After surgery I was very depressed. I had known of the pregnancy less than twenty-four hours before surgery. Yet neither my doctors nor the nurses tried to get me to talk about how I was feeling. They treated it just as if it were 'another operation,' but it had a lot more meaning to me — I lost a chance to have a baby."

As you were recovering from the surgery, you begin to realize what has happened to you. In a short period of time, you experienced a life-threatening medical condition, lost a pregnancy, and lost one of your fallopian tubes. So much has happened that your head may be reeling and you may feel unable to assimilate it all. In addition, your initial feeling that you were lucky to survive has probably started to pale, and the specter of what you have lost now seems enormous.

PHYSICAL RECOVERY

Because you may have had severe pain and bleeding, perhaps even hemorrhage, and because you have had major surgery involving anesthesia and medication, physical recovery from an ectopic pregnancy can take a month, possibly longer. It is important to get a lot of rest during this time.

Most physicians prefer to do a physical examination two to three weeks following surgery. During this visit, your doctor is likely to discuss your surgery in detail and inform you of its implications for future pregnancies.

If you are having no physical problems and your incision is healing well, your physician will probably give you permission to have sexual intercourse. However, he will probably suggest that you wait until you have had three normal menstrual cycles before you attempt to become pregnant again, and that you use a mechanical method of birth control (diaphragm, condom, foam) during this time.

THE EMOTIONAL AFTERMATH

Not until you had been home for a while did the full impact of your loss strike you. You have just been through a life-threatening crisis. You realize now that you could have died. You lost your pregnancy, perhaps after years of trying to conceive. You've found out that your chances for a successful pregnancy are dismal.

Added to all this is the problem that most people don't seem to understand what you're going through. You may have chosen not to tell anyone you had an ectopic pregnancy. If you told friends and relatives, it is possible that they discuss it as a surgical procedure when it is much more than that to you. They may think as long as you have "one good side," it will make little difference. But you know what your doctor has said and it scares you — your chances of having a baby are reduced and the likelihood that you will have another ectopic pregnancy is significant.

If you have other children, they may have been around during the emergency, seen you in acute pain, and not been able to understand the cause. Then you were rushed to the hospital, where you stayed for up to a week. It might have been the first time you were separated from them for this length of time. There lives have been disrupted and it's been a traumatic period for them. Try to stay close to them so they will not feel shut out.

During the aftermath, you will probably go through times of vulnerability, bewilderment, anger, guilt, jealousy, and grief if you are like the women we counseled.

Vulnerability

It is common to feel extremely vulnerable after having an ectopic pregnancy. It may have been the first time your own life has been endangered. Your concern was not just about the baby's death, but the possibility of your own. Perhaps for the first time you had a sense of how fragile life is, how little control we have. You were lucky; they caught it in time — you didn't die and there were no complications, but the threat existed and is frightening to think of.

Bewilderment

So much has happened so quickly that you may feel completely bewildered. You were perplexed at the time when it was going on and you find that you remain puzzled as you try to sort things out.

Kathy, in her mid-twenties, expressed her confusion as follows: "I was very sad and felt a death had occurred. I felt empty and puzzled as to *why*. I comforted myself by thinking it was an early pregnancy and realizing it would have been harder to lose a baby later, as with stillbirth. I fell back on the thought that I had gotten pregnant after years of infertility. All told, my thoughts and emotions were mixed, sometimes conflicting and sometimes disturbing."

Anger

It is common to feel furious that an ectopic pregnancy happened to you. You didn't deserve it. You want a baby so badly and you are frustrated because it doesn't seem as if you'll ever have one. You realize your anger is irrational, but you feel it nonetheless. At times you are certain it was no one's fault and other times you question whether it was. Why wasn't it discovered earlier? you ponder angrily; maybe then the damage wouldn't be so bad.

As a young secretary said: "I was 'mad at the world' at times after the loss of my pregnancy and my left tube. I was astonished at my occasional anger with some little thing that went wrong. I couldn't seem to control it. I realized I felt frustrated and didn't know what to do about it. I talked it over with my husband and he understood better why I was so irritable. I felt I needed to talk about my feelings with women who had gone through something similar, so I joined a discussion group I heard about through a friend. This helped me the most because we shared our feelings and learned we weren't neurotic — that our emotions were understandable considering the circumstances. We also helped each other cope."

Many women are disturbed by the scars of an ectopic pregnancy, both mental and physical. The physical scar is not pretty to look at, but that's not really what bothers you the most. What is most upsetting is that the scar reminds you of your loss.

Blame and Guilt

You may find it hard to accept the fact that your tubal pregnancy "just happened." You feel a compulsion to find out whose fault it was and to blame someone or something for causing it.

Frequently, women blame their doctors for causing the ectopic pregnancy or failing to diagnose it early. There may be times when a doctor makes a mistake, and that is unfortunate. There are many more times, however, when the tubal pregnancy could not have been diagnosed any earlier than it was.

You may blame your doctor for failing to save your tube when it was unsalvageable. Your feelings and need to place blame may get in the way of rational thought. People tend to feel angry at the doctor who "mutilated" them, as one woman termed it.

Possibly, you blame yourself for what happened. Women commonly feel guilty for things that happened in the past, thinking that "I brought it on myself." They can't forgive themselves for undergoing reconstructive surgery on their tubes despite the risks, or having contracted venereal disease years earlier. While feeling guilty serves no constructive purpose and makes you feel worse, it is difficult to let go of the idea that you are being punished for your sins.

Envy

You may envy women who are pregnant or those who have healthy children. Feeling jealous is a common reaction. It doesn't seem fair that those around you are easily having babies and you envy their good luck. You may feel sad every time you see a pregnant woman or a baby and find yourself consciously trying to avoid such encounters whenever possible.

Grief and Mourning

With ectopic pregnancy, there is likely to be grief and sadness on many levels. The couple mourns not only the loss of the pregnancy, but also the possibility that their fertility has been reduced. The couple with a history of infertility prior to the ectopic pregnancy is not unusual. This couple is particularly apt to feel a double sense of loss when a pregnancy fails because it was a long-awaited and extremely precious pregnancy.

Toby, in her early thirties, describes her terrible sense of loss following a tubal pregnancy after difficulty in conceiving. "I felt sure, after fifteen long months of anxiety, tests, and waiting, that I was finally pregnant. Then it just didn't seem possible that I was going into surgery that was to take away the baby I had prayed and longed for.

"I felt such a tremendous sense of loss and emptiness, and to top that, I felt the discomfort that follows surgery. The real depression occurred when I got home and the full impact of what happened was felt. Not only was I cheated out of a baby, but how could I ever have another one with only one fallopian tube, my husband's low sperm count, and my irregular ovulation?

"To me, the odds were overwhelmingly against me. For weeks I'd find myself crying for that lost baby that I was never given a chance to feel or know."

For Toby and many others, losing a pregnancy was extremely painful. They experienced many of the emotions common to early pregnancy loss described in Part I. In addition, their feelings of grief were often compounded by feelings about the loss or reduction of fertility which resulted from the ectopic pregnancy.

With ectopic pregnancy you may grieve less for the actual baby, since you knew you were pregnant for such a short time, if you knew at all, than for the lost opportunity, your lost fertility. Sandy describes her delayed grief: "Since I didn't even know I was pregnant, the whole thing seemed like emergency surgery and not much more. Then, later, it hit me that I had lost a baby. However, I felt the most anxiety when it sank in that my chances of having a successful pregnancy in the future were much lower."

Meredith had similar feelings and commented on the impact her tubal pregnancy had on her life. "I only knew for a few days that I was pregnant so I didn't have time to get very excited. But we had been trying to have a baby for eighteen months, so I did get excited for a few days and was terribly disappointed the way things turned out. I felt very badly in the months that followed the loss. It is only lately that I have been gradually improving; there is still much depression and despair. Occasionally, I have had mild suicidal impulses. We have wanted a child for so long and we have no idea what the future holds. With one tube gone, I know my chances of getting pregnant are less, and I have an increased chance of another ectopic pregnancy. That absolutely terrifies me. I grew up thinking of pregnancy as a wonderful time, and now that has been ruined."

After an ectopic pregnancy it is necessary to heal both physically and emotionally. Fortunately the process of physical recovery is almost always uneventful and is usually accomplished within a month or two. Emotional recovery tends to occur more gradually as one comes to terms with what has happened, and as one assesses what one has lost and what is still possible.

Many women have found that the support and understanding of friends and family were invaluable in helping them along this road. If it is at all possible, talk to others who share your experience. They have a special knowledge of what you have been through. These conversations should convince you that you are not alone, that your feelings are comprehensible, and that other women have felt the way you have and have managed to pick up the pieces of their lives and go on. This can be both a solace and an inspiration.

They have made it and you can. The natural course of grief is one of gradual healing. There are also things you can do to speed your recovery. Anything that reconnects you to life helps: seeing friends, working, socializing, to name a few. Do not be discouraged if at first it takes an effort to do these things. Each step along the way should be easier than the one before it.

THE HUSBAND'S EXPERIENCE

Your husband is likely to have many of the same emotional reactions to the ectopic pregnancy as you have had. He, too, will be affected by the pregnancy loss because he wanted a child also, and by the knowledge that his chances of becoming a father are diminished.

Yet your husband's concern about losing the pregnancy and decreased fertility are probably overshadowed by his fear of losing you. When you pulled through, the fact that you survived was utmost in his mind. He may seem less upset than you are about losing the baby. It's not that he didn't want the baby; it's just that he was terribly worried about you and feels grateful you are all right.

Most men develop an attachment to their unborn child later in the pregnancy than their wives do. With ectopic pregnancy, this attachment may not have developed at all, since the pregnancy terminated so early. In fact, your husband may not have even known you were pregnant. Within the span of a few hours he may have been confronted with the news that you were pregnant, that you were being rushed to the operating room for emergency surgery, and that you would lose the pregnancy. That's a great deal for him to handle all at once. He, too, was probably shocked and had to deal with his own feelings of bewilderment and pain as well as yours.

Men and women generally perceive pregnancy differently, so the chances are that your husband coped with the pregnancy loss, surgery, and implications for fertility in a different way from yours. For a better understanding of the discrepancies in the experience for husbands and wives, we suggest you read the section on the marital relationship.

WHAT CAUSES ECTOPIC PREGNANCY?

In about half the cases of ectopic pregnancy, no cause is found. The most common causes of interference with the progress of the fertilized ovum are damage to the tube from chronic pelvic inflammatory disease (usually secondary to gonorrhea and, rarely, associated with postabortion infection), previous pelvic surgery, or a prior ectopic pregnancy or reconstructive surgery (tubo-plasty).

Other conditions thought to be causes are developmental abnor-malities of the tube such as excessive length, diverticula involving outpouching of the tube and kinking, obstruction from sources outside the tube itself, and hormonal factors that affect the trans-port of the egg through the tube. At the present time there is some evidence that women who have used an IUD (intrauterine device) may have a higher incidence of ectopic pregnancy than might oth-erwise be expected. However, further studies need to be done be-fore this has been definitively determined.

GETTING ON WITH YOUR LIFE

It was bad enough to lose the baby after trying hard to get preg-nant, but the final blow came when your doctor told you that there was even more to be concerned about. If it was your first ectopic pregnancy and you have one tube left, your chance of getting pregnant again may be diminished. Only 50 percent of women conceive after having had an ectopic pregnancy. In addition, there is an increased chance that there may be something wrong with your remaining tube, for whatever caused the problem with your first tube (such as obstructed tubes because of pelvic inflammatory disease, tubal surgery, or other infection) may also have affected your remaining tube. Subsequently, the woman who has suffered one ectopic pregnancy has an increased risk, 7 to 12 percent, de-pending on the study, of having a second.

If your tube had previously been removed (this may be your sec-ond ectopic pregnancy) or you know it is badly damaged or mal-formed, it is highly possible that your fertility may be grossly im-paired or completely absent.

When the initial shock has worn off and you are feeling better physically, you can begin putting things into perspective. One thing is clear: becoming a parent will be no simple matter. You have a long, hard road ahead of you. For a while, you'll need to assimilate what has happened and you will need to grieve. When you feel ready, you will deal with what to do next: get another medical opinion, try to conceive again, undergo reconstructive surgery, adopt.

It is best to enter into the decision-making process after you understand your medical condition completely — what you lost and what you have left. It is then that you can look at your alternatives and consider which is best for you.

(1) If you have potential fertility, you must decide whether to try to get pregnant again. In doing so, you may be risking another ectopic pregnancy, however.

(2) If you have had conservative surgery that salvaged your damaged tube, or if you have tubal obstruction on the opposite side, you need to decide if you want to undergo reconstructive surgery. When successful, this surgery should improve your chances of conceiving. However, one unfortunate consequence of the surgery in some women, is that scarring resulting from the tubal surgery may increase the possibility that another ectopic pregnancy may occur.

(3) If you are infertile, as a consequence of having lost both tubes or because your tubal damage is too extensive for reconstructive surgery to be helpful, the choices that remain to you are adoption or childlessness.

For those who are potentially fertile and decide to try again, it still remains to be seen whether or not Nature will do her part. When conception does not occur, there are many stresses to contend with. Among these may be diagnostic tests to assess whether or not you have an open fallopian tube or tubes, basal body temperature charts to maximize your chances of getting pregnant, months of eager anticipation followed by crushing disappointment, and maybe even reconstructive surgery to repair a damaged tube. If conception occurs quickly, one hurdle is passed, and the anxious waiting begins. Only when it has been definitely established that the pregnancy is intrauterine is it possible to breathe a sigh of relief.

If your problem is not one of uncertain fertility, but one of definite sterility, this must be dealt with. Under the best of circumstances, it is extremely difficult to make peace with the loss of your capacity to reproduce. However, when you feel robbed of your fertility by an accident of nature, or by the unforeseen consequences of your own actions, the loss may be even more difficult to accept.

Infertility resulting from an ectopic pregnancy is both an insult and an assault, because it both damages your sense of wholeness, thus threatening your psychological wellbeing, and causes you bodily harm as well. The dual nature of the assault complicates the grieving process. Not only must one mourn the loss of fertility; the loss of one's body wholeness must be coped with, too.

Despite the fact that your options are clear, you may feel confused and unable to make a decision. This is a common reaction after ectopic pregnancy. After all, this has been a major life crisis and it may take a long time before you recover. You have had to come to terms with the issue of death — no simple task for *anyone.* Often, people who have been traumatized by a recent brush with death have trouble in making decisions. It may help you to know that one day everything will fall into place and you will find your choice clear.

One Woman's Story

We were sitting in a cafe with friends on a Sunday afternoon when I felt the first pains. My heart sank — cramps, I thought, even though my temperature hadn't dropped at all that morning. I gazed at the chart of my basal temperature several times every day like some ancient priestess trying to divine the future by observing the flight of birds. I had been taking my temperature for four months as part of the fertility workup my gynecologist was conducting. For a year now I had greeted each new cycle with the hope that this time I would become pregnant, and every time the menstrual flow began I experienced increasing disappointment and frustration. This time I had watched the days pass, ritually acknowledged every morning on the chart — 28, 29, 30. . . . I became more hopeful and more excited. And now, I was sitting, talking with friends, outwardly calm and cheerful, but inwardly terribly sad. I didn't feel any flow beginning, but that was usual for me. Cramps could signal the beginning of the menstrual flow several hours before it began in earnest. But I was very surprised and confused when I got home several hours later and still found no flow. But the cramps persisted.

Monday morning the thermometer registered 99°. The cramps and the continuing absence of menstrual flow had me puzzled. I so much wanted to believe that the temperature chart meant that I was pregnant, but my body seemed to be telling me otherwise. I debated inwardly for a while, and then called my doctor. It turned out that he was out of town attending a conference, and I was put through to the physician who was taking his cases. I described my situation and current symptoms, but the doctor didn't think they warranted an office visit.

Tuesday morning my temperature was over 99°. Since 99° was the highest number on the chart, I drew the line up above the chart to approximately where I thought the next degree markings would go. The chart was still my oracle, but not a very interpretable one. I could never get my temperature line to go in the neat ups and downs of the illustration. Staying up late, having a glass of wine, or sleeping in late all would affect the temperature reading.

I was not working at the time. I had quit my job half because I wanted time off and half because I optimistically expected to be pregnant. I offered my help at a little theater some friends of ours were starting up. On that Tuesday morning I still had cramps and was glad I was scheduled to work as rehearsal assistant because I thought that activity would take my mind off my discomfort and distract me from my growing uneasiness about the meaning of the pain. Halfway through the rehearsal the pain became so intense that I couldn't sit upright in my chair. I apologetically told a friend that I had to leave. She took one look at my face, white and beaded with sweat, and whisked me off home.

Of the number of things I learned during the whole frightening process of the ectopic pregnancy, one of the most important for me has been how to present myself to physicians when I need medical help. I grew up in a family in which stoicism and the unflinching endurance of pain were main values. I accepted without question that the appropriate behavior, no matter how intense the pain, was calmly to describe the problem to the doctor and wait for him to help me. My regular gynecologist knew me fairly well, and he recognised this feature of my character (we talked about it after the whole experience was over). But the physician taking his place had no such background knowledge of me, and he based his judgments on his experience with his patients in general.

This time, when I called, the doctor said to come right in, and he squeezed in time between two scheduled patients to see me. I came into the examination room clutching my temperature chart in my hand and holding myself carefully upright. I calmly described my symptoms to him, and then he examined me. Then he said it was unclear what was going on. I might be pregnant, but it was too soon to tell. Sometimes pregnancy produced puzzling symptoms, like pain, but it couldn't be an ectopic pregnancy, because I didn't have enough pain. And what, I inquired quietly, constituted enough pain? Pain so intense that women scream and roll around, he said.

I was dumbfounded. I could not begin to explain that I could not imagine a circumstance that would cause me to act like that. When I was a teenager, my mother fell down while hiking and broke her leg in two places. My father carried her to a fire road, and from there she was evacuated by jeep. She never screamed or rolled around, although it was clear that she was in considerable pain. The pain the doctor was describing was clearly outside my realm of experience, and my *pain did not qualify as a major symptom. As I left the doctor's office I was aware of being deeply embarrassed. I had committed an unforgivable sin — I had acted like a hysterical female.*

My husband had taken me to my appointment, and as we drove home I passed on the doctor's assurance that I was all right because I didn't have enough pain for it to be an ectopic pregnancy. He didn't know exactly what an ectopic pregnancy was, so when we got home I drew him a picture of the ovaries, tubes, and uterus. He was relieved that that was not the problem, but since he could see that I was still uncomfortable, he asked if maybe I should go see our internist. The covering doctor had suggested that my symptoms might not be the result of a gynecological problem, but I was still so embarrassed at crying wolf that I refused to consult another physician.

I passed the rest of that day and night in a fog of ambiguity. What did the pain mean? Was I pregnant and about to miscarry? Was I just having a difficult period? Did I have a strange form of appendicitis in which the pain appeared on the left side instead of the right? I tried to get my mind off my pain and my worry. But no sooner would I succeed in distracting myself than I would find my attention going back to my abdomen. Had the pain diminished? Yes, it did seem less than before; no, wait a minute, that was quite a strong twinge — and on and on.

Except for my doctor, no one knew that we were trying to have a baby. At first, I had just wanted to present my friends and family with a fait accompli. I had thought that I would be pregnant within a few months of deciding I wanted to be. Then, as the months drew on and nothing happened, I became even more reticent about telling anyone. I feared there was something wrong with me — something very deeply wrong — and I didn't want anyone to know. So now during the days of ambiguity I had no one, except my husband, with whom to share my fear and my longing. My husband was, as always, my mainstay. He took care of me, and kept track of how I was feeling. But even he did not understand my deep longing for a baby, and so could not share my emotions. Not until the doctor finally gave a definite diagnosis and I was being wheeled into surgery did he grasp the meaning of the loss.

Wednesday morning, my temperature went up another notch. I was half joyful, half despairing. In the months before, the line on the chart had taken that long plunge that indicated the onset of menstruation, and my hopes had plunged with my temperature. So part of me still hoped that I might be pregnant, and everything would be all right. But another part of my mind thought that at least if my temperature dropped, I would have some clarity about what was going on. I almost began to hope that it would drop, that the bleeding would start and I would have some resolution.

During the morning the pain became more and more intense. I must have picked up the phone fifteen times to call the doctor, but each time I put it down again. How much pain was enough? *I didn't want to risk feeling like a fool again. Finally, around midday I was overwhelmed by a sharp, intense, sickening pain. This had to be enough pain. I lay on the sofa, too ill even to get to the telephone. Then the pain subsided. I felt better. Good thing I hadn't called the doctor, I thought, or he'd really have me pegged as a hypochondriac.*

My husband called in the middle of the afternoon to see how I was doing, and was greatly relieved when I told him that I had had a lot of pain in the morning, but it had now all gone away. Although I didn't know it at the time, that intense pain was the tube "blowing" (to use the doctor's word). The tiny embryo that had somehow implanted in my tube and found enough nourishment to grow had burst the fallopian tube. So I was happy in my ignorance that afternoon, and cheerfully went about doing chores I had neglected for the past few days, not knowing that all the while I was bleeding internally and that in a short time I was about to experience "enough" pain.

The first twinges definitely felt like cramps. I went upstairs and took my temperature again, even though it was late afternoon. I still had a low-grade fever. Could I have some infection that was causing the fever and masking the usual drop before my period? I was again swamped in ambiguity.

I felt some nausea by evening and didn't eat much dinner. I left the table before my husband had finished eating, and went upstairs to lie down. He soon followed me worriedly into our bedroom. In the next hours, as the pain increased and I found it impossible to read or distract myself in any way, he kept pacing around and checking on me. He tried to get me to call the doctor. I didn't want to bother the doctor at home, I told him. When he said he was going to call, I yelled at him, and then cried. We called the doctor.

As before, I spoke to the doctor calmly and quietly. I described my symptoms in detail. He prescribed codeine, and my husband went to an all-night pharmacy to get it. I awaited his return impatiently. At last, something to relieve the pain. I might then begin to be able to think straight and extricate myself from this web of fear and pain.

The codeine upset my stomach. I stumbled into the bathroom to vomit, and realized that I felt very faint. My husband half carried me back to the bedroom. I could neither stand nor sit up without blacking out. I lay on the bed writhing in pain and moaning. My husband called the doctor back and described what was going on. I was too ill to talk. My husband had no personal rules about telling the doctor in unemotional tones what was going on. He conveyed his worry and concern. The doctor said he would meet us at the hospital.

The trip to the hospital had all the elements of slapstick comedy. Had I not been so sick I would surely have protested. I live two blocks from the hospital. But since I could neither stand nor walk, and since my husband couldn't carry me down the stairs to the car, he called an ambulance. As it turned out, their stretcher couldn't fit down our stairs, so the men ended up carrying me. The ambulance attendant called me "honey" and regaled me with stories of other people he had transported that night (the one right before me had a gunshot wound). My husband rode in the front and gave the driver directions — he didn't know how to get to the hospital.

Once we arrived at the emergency room, there began what seemed like an endless series of examinations. By this time, the accumulated blood in the abdominal cavity was causing spasms in all the abdominal muscles, and the pressure of the blood on the diaphragm caused referred pain in my upper chest. The merest touch could set off these incredibly painful spasms, and it seemed as if people never stopped poking, prodding, pushing, and feeling. My husband squeezed my hand and stroked my head while I cried and begged them to stop. Finally I heard myself screaming.

At long last, they stopped and I was left alone with my husband while they awaited the results of some blood tests. I felt sure that I was dying, and I wanted to tell my husband how much he meant to me, and what a good life we had had together. I was searching for the words, but he was already on another tack. If the doctor didn't come up with anything definite, he said, he was going to call our internist. They weren't sure it was a gynecological problem anyway. The doctor came back in and said that the tests were inconclusive and that they were going to put me under observation. The doctor's announcement sent me into despair. This was it, I thought; they were just going to watch me die. My husband went out into the hall with the doctor and came back to tell me that they had called our internist.

It wasn't my regular internist who arrived, though, but one of his associates, whom I had never met. He was a young man who immediately dispensed with any pretense at a bedside manner. I later forgave him because he quickly got to the root of the matter, but at the time it was a little disconcerting. The other doctors had been very kind and concerned, apologizing for hurting me. This one began with a series of accusatory questions — what drugs had I been taking; how much did I drink? He acted as if he knew that I was a dope-fiend alcoholic. His certainty convinced even me. I confessed that I did usually have a glass of wine with dinner.

When he began to examine me, I could feel another painful spasm starting. I knew that if he touched me, it would start up an agonizing series of spasms. As he reached out his hand, I grabbed him by the wrist with all the strength I could muster. He gave me a startled look. I could see that I had scared him. It must be an unwritten rule that the doctor touches the patient, but the patient does not touch the doctor.

Then he was in charge of the situation again. His examination was quick and incredibly gentle — not what his manner had led me to expect. Then he took my blood pressure. They must have taken my blood pressure a hundred times since I had been admitted. He left the blood pressure cuff on my arm and told me to sit up. I told him that I couldn't, that I passed out when I sat up. He just put his arm behind me and hauled me into a sitting position, and took my blood pressure again while everything slowly went black before my eyes. He lowered me again. Then he placed his stethoscope on my abdomen and with two fingers pushed down as far as he could and let go suddenly. I could see my abdomen rise first on the right side, then on the left, as the fluid inside sloshed back and forth.

These two tests seemed to clinch it for him. He went into a huddle with the gynecologist, and then the quiet room was bustling with activity. No one told me anything. Suddenly, I was swept over with the most exquisite sensation of relief. It was as if someone had taken a magical eraser and wiped the pain from my body. They had just given me intravenous Demerol. They had their diagnosis; they no longer needed my pain as a guide. Then the final test — a needle through the abdominal wall to see if there was blood in the abdominal cavity. There was.

Things happened quickly after that. My husband had stayed by my side throughout the ordeal. At the doors to the operating room we had to part. I panicked. I fought against the drug-induced euphoria. Now I had to say something, because I might not make it through. "I love you, I love you" was all I could think to say. He kissed me, and then I was wheeled into the operating room.

The anesthesiologist was immediately by my side, introducing himself and asking if I were allergic to any drugs. All the while he was rigging up an apparatus, and introducing another needle into my arm. I could see that I would be out cold in a matter of seconds. I asked where the doctor was, and pleaded with the anesthesiologist to wait before he put me out. I was told the doctor was preparing for surgery and would be along in a minute, but they had to go ahead with their preparations.

The anesthesiologist began to inject the sodium pentothal. "Give him a message from me, please," I begged. The doctor slowed down his injection. I was beginning to fade. "Tell him to be conservative," and then I was out. I went down fighting for control of the situation, and desperately afraid that the doctor might not try to salvage what he could of my reproductive organs. No one had told me what the surgery would consist of — I thought I might wake up to find I had had a hysterectomy.

The next few days run together for me. They are not a blur, but rather a series of vivid scenes. From this point on, everything that had to do with pregnancy or babies was very highly charged for me. The loss of the embryo and the loss of the tube made me even more obsessed with becoming pregnant, but initially I was sunk in grief. I found reminders everywhere.

I woke up in the intensive care unit because the recovery room was not yet open. I was definitely in the way there, and I heard grumbling around me. They sent a maternity nurse down to take care of me. Once in my hospital room, I found that one of my roommates had had a hysterectomy. The other was an eighteen-year-old girl who already had two children and was in the hospital for an abortion.

My husband came late in the morning. He had stayed outside the operating room until the surgery was completed. He had talked to the doctor, and then gone home to sleep. He told me he had been overwhelmed when he realized that there had been a tiny baby — part of him and part of me. Up till then, our efforts at pregnancy had somehow seemed theoretical to him. But now, too late, he grasped the reality, and the loss seemed awful.

Calling my parents and telling them was very hard. My mother had been planning to visit, and she advanced her time of arrival to coincide with my getting out of the hospital. I'll never forget the shocked look on her face when she saw me get out of the car on my homecoming day. Acting in the family tradition, I had played down my illness to her. Her face told me better than any mirror how ghastly I looked.

The doctors had decided not to transfuse me because they had recently had problems with the current supply of blood — people had been contracting hepatitis. So I was supplied with iron pills and a diet that included red meat twice a day. The anemia, however, was one of the hardest things I had to deal with. It took me a couple of months to build myself up again, and the inability to do anything without sweating, panting, and feeling exhausted added greatly to my depression.

I quickly got back into the fertility workup, though. The doctor advised a certain period of time for recovery from surgery, and then I was again taking my temperature every morning, and having intercourse on prescribed days at prescribed times. I cross-examined the doctor on the probability of a second ectopic, and we set out a plan for how to deal with it if I even suspected I might be having a second one. I found out that there is an association between infertility and ectopic pregnancies. But I was also assured that many women bear full-term babies after having an ectopic pregnancy. I lived with the hope.

Six months later the doctor recommended that I see a specialist. He summed up his findings and said that the evidence was inconclusive as to what was wrong. His best guess was that something was not quite right with the remaining tube. On the other hand, he said, it might be something else too subtle for his tests to pick up. I told the doctor that I needed a break, and he agreed that this might be a good thing.

It is one of the ironic conditions of life that the anxiety to become pregnant can act to interfere with impregnation. I hoped that if I could get away from the daily fascination of the temperature chart and the monthly timing of intercourse, I might achieve through relaxation what I couldn't through science. By this time my relationship with my husband was under strain. I was obsessed with becoming pregnant, and our sexual life had lost all spontaneity. When we visited friends of ours who had a new baby, I would be fine during the visit, then sob all the way home in the car.

In addition, I was haunted by memories of the ectopic pregnancy. I couldn't shake the horrifying memories of those days of pain. It could hit me almost anytime, but particularly in that time of going to sleep, when the conscious guards are down, I would suddenly be thrown back into the nightmare, reliv-

ing it second by second. Then I would turn my face into the pillow and cry. My husband would hold me and try to comfort me. He didn't understand what was going on, but he was infinitely patient with me.

So I called a halt to the further pursuit of infertility consultations, and I entered graduate school to prepare myself for a new career. Too much idle time was grist for the mill of depression. I threw myself into my work, and derived considerable satisfaction from it and from the new friends I made. But nearly a year and a half after the ectopic pregnancy I realized that I was still reliving the terror. This was not healthy, I decided, and I started seeing a therapist. She helped me tremendously. I dealt with and got rid of the waking nightmare. It became an experience of the past, instead of one I relived constantly in the present. And I dealt with my own deep fears about there being something wrong with me because I wasn't able to become pregnant.

My time spent in therapy was a tremendous liberation for me. Freed from the shackles of fear and bad feelings about myself, I could begin to think in a new light about having a child. I was no longer obsessed with pregnancy. I wanted a child very, very much, but my whole sense of myself as being all right did not depend upon it.

I went to see the specialist my gynecologist recommended. He concurred with my physician. There was most likely something wrong with my remaining tube. Surgery might be able to correct it. If it could be surgically corrected, he would give me a 30 percent chance of pregnancy. I was not impressed by the odds. I cried all the way home.

I talked it over with my husband, and thought about it a lot myself. If I had the surgery and if the tube could be repaired, there was still no guarantee of pregnancy. I remembered the months of the reign of the thermometer and the scheduled intercourse, the waiting anxiously every thirty days, the depression and the despair.

One weekend while I was still debating with myself about the surgery, I had an experience that made up my mind for me. I was gardening in my front yard. A little girl who lives several houses away was trying to learn to ride her two-wheeler. She could go a few yards before she fell over. She fell near where I was weeding, and I helped her up and then spent some time holding her bicycle straight and pushing her while she strove to get the feeling of balance. All the while, as usually happened whenever I was around children, I was filled with an intense longing to have children of my own to love and care for and help learn to ride bicycles. Then it hit me. I looked at the little girl and realized — I could love this child. She doesn't have my genes or my hus-

band's. She doesn't look like either of us, but I could love her as if she were my own. Here I had been spending all my time thinking only of pregnancy. What I wanted was a baby.

That was the turning point. What happened next is truly another story. Briefly, I'll say that we pursued an independent adoption, and within a year we were holding a beautiful, healthy baby boy in our arms and bringing him home. As I write this now, we are on the eve of our day in court when the adoption will become legal. We are very pleased to have all the legal proceedings complete, but from the moment we first held him in our arms we knew he was our baby.

It took four weeks from conception for the embryo to burst the fallopian tube. It took four years from the ectopic pregnancy to reach the decision to adopt. I now have accepted the loss of the baby that might have been and the loss of my own reproductive function, but I know that, for me, it took a long time.

5. Multiple Losses — When It Happens Again

When you lost your first pregnancy everyone told you not to worry — it happens to a lot of people. "Remember you are young and healthy and have lots of time to have babies," they all said. And you believed them, or at least you tried to.

It is hard to say when you began to believe that maybe they were wrong. If you have not been able to become pregnant again, or if you have and have lost these pregnancies too — chances are you are not as hopeful as you once were. You ask yourself if you really want to keep trying and when is the time to stop.

Other women seem to have babies so easily; why not you? Lightning is not supposed to strike twice in the same place, and certainly not three times — or four times. Why is this happening to you? you ask. You've suffered enough; you've paid your dues; you want a baby more than anything else in the world. It just isn't fair.

After a while you feel convinced that there is something wrong with you, that you will never have the child you want. You feel damaged and incomplete. Sometimes you feel so frustrated you could scream; some days you cannot shake your feelings of despair. You blame yourself; you blame the world. You hate yourself for envying other women and because having a baby is so important to you. You can't help noticing that your obsession with having a baby is taking a toll on you, on your family, and perhaps even on your friendships. You want to go on with life — to have all of this behind you — but there doesn't seem to be an end in sight.

The loss of a pregnancy is always painful, no matter if you have lost two pregnancies or ten. Consciously you may try not to be too hopeful, so as to protect yourself from disappointment if something does go wrong. Nevertheless, you can't help but feel disappointed if your pregnancy ends.

Most couples report that they have experienced increasing difficulty coping with each succeeding loss. Not only does one experience grief and mourning anew every time; eventually one starts to question whether something is seriously wrong and whether it will ever be possible to produce a child. In order that feelings of despair, hopelessness, frustration, jealousy, anger and worthlessness not dominate one's life it is necessary to mourn each loss completely. Unfortunately, this becomes harder and harder to do, because as the blows accumulate, it is harder to put them behind you and your resources for doing so work less well. Some couples have found that their ability to recover disappeared completely at some point, and that although the acute pain diminished, they were left with persistent and unshakable feelings of depression. This was described variously as feeling that life had become "dead," that it was hard to enjoy things, and difficult to feel excited by anything. Often despair looms so large that it takes over everything — every part of life is overshadowed by the pain.

Lisa and John sought counseling help after their third miscarriage because they felt that their attempts to deal with their difficulties on their own had not been successful. Lisa, a talented lawyer, had quit her job with a large law firm after her second miscarriage in the hopes that a less pressured existence would permit her to carry a pregnancy successfully. After three months of trying to conceive, she became pregnant. After two blissful months of pregnancy, she began to spot, and eventually miscarried. Both Lisa and John were devastated. They felt that they had done everything in their power to make this pregnancy successful. They felt helpless to do anything differently or better next time, and with this realization they felt totally at a loss. Lisa found that she was unable to think of anything else besides getting pregnant, being pregnant, and staying pregnant. She started to find it increasingly difficult to do anything outside the house, and for the first time in her life she even avoided friends. She felt acutely envious of several who had children, and found even telephone conversations with them agonizing. Worst of all, she was unable to tell anyone but John what was wrong. She had been raised to believe that she should keep her troubles to herself, lest other people think badly of her. Even though the isolation she was imposing on herself was unbearable, the thought that her friends or family would know how unsuccessful she was was even more painful. John, on the other hand, got to hear every detail of her experiences, over and over again. Although he felt totally sympathetic and, in fact, shared her feelings, he found that a constant diet of grief was more than he could bear. He felt at a loss in remedying the situation, especially after they visited several new doctors, who found nothing conclusive. His decision to seek couples' counseling was reached when he recognized that not only was Lisa not getting over her grief; rather, she was becoming increasingly depressed and so was he.

Although they did not realize it at the time, both John and Lisa had been behaving in ways that were unproductive but that gave them some measure of control over what had happened to them: Lisa blamed herself instead of blaming fate, and John kept trying to make things better, despite the fact that there wasn't anything he or anyone else could do. These behavior patterns were not successful because they prevented the couple from coming to terms with the fact that sometimes in life things happen for no apparent reason and sometimes one is powerless to change them.

In therapy Lisa was able to separate her feelings about herself from her feelings about losing the pregnancies. She had originally experienced her miscarriages as tangible evidence of how inadequate she really was. Eventually, she came to recognize that although many unfortunate things had happened to her, this did not mean that she was bad or worthless. Once these feelings were resolved, she felt freer to let people know what she was going through, and to ask for their support. In addition, she began to enjoy life again and to recapture her optimism about the future.

Like Lisa, John discovered that he could not always be responsible for everything that happened. This realization allowed him to feel less helpless when he was unable to improve things. He was surprised to find that as he was more able to tolerate his own grief, his empathy for Lisa grew, thereby strengthening their relationship.

John's and Lisa's situation is not unique. Although not everyone reacts the way they did, it is common to find that one's feelings about the actual loss are compounded by doubts, fears, or misgivings about oneself. These need to be dealt with so that needed energy is not diverted from the challenge at hand.

Why is it that, although most couples have no difficulty having a baby, some have so much? Doctors are not sure of how to answer this question, because although they know a great deal about why some couples have difficulty conceiving, and about why others lose their pregnancies, there is a lot that they don't know as yet.

If you have lost two or more pregnancies, or if you have been unable to become pregnant again after six months to a year of trying, your physician probably has suggested that you have a complete medical evaluation to determine the source of your difficulty. This evaluation may provide you with an explanation of why you have been having problems. There may be things that your physician can do to correct whatever may have been wrong. However, it may be that even a thorough medical evaluation will not succeed in turning up the source of your difficulties. As you know, it is often impossible to explain what caused a given miscarriage, stillbirth, or ectopic pregnancy. There is also much that is not known about why some couples experience multiple losses: repeated miscarriages, repeated stillbirths, or several ectopic pregnancies; or some combination of these. Similarly, more often than not, the reason why some women are unable to conceive, after having done so at least once, cannot be determined.

How long to keep trying is a highly individual decision. Many couples do finally succeed in having a child after numerous losses. Others have chosen to give up, some after one or two losses and others after many attempts. Still others have lost several pregnancies, then produced a child, later had more losses, and eventually produced more children.

Each couple must decide for themselves how much they can handle. Some things to think about in making this decision are: is there a known cause of our difficulties? If so, is there a specific treatment available, and what is the likelihood that it will be successful? If not, what is the likelihood that future attempts at pregnancy will be met with success? Also, can you cope with another pregnancy, and perhaps another disappointment? Alternatively, can you face giving up? Lastly, you need to think about alternatives such as adoption or childless living and decide if either of these is a choice you wish to make at the present time.

HABITUAL ABORTION

A concern commonly voiced by couples who have had a miscarriage is "What are the chances that our next pregnancy will be successful?" If you have not had more than one or two miscarriages, the answer to this question is quite encouraging. After one or two miscarriages, the statistical risk of having another is about the same as the risk of having one in the first place. This is because, in all likelihood, each was caused by random, unrelated events that have little likelihood of recurring.

A woman is said to be a "habitual aborter" if she has had three or more consecutive pregnancies that have terminated in miscarriage. Whether each of the miscarriages was caused by random factors or whether they were caused by recurrent, underlying difficulty must be assessed for each individual.

Studies of women who have had three consecutive miscarriages without a live birth have found that the chance that a fourth pregnancy will result in a live birth is somewhere between 20 percent and 80 percent. This range is too wide to be of help in predicting what the outcome of a particular woman's pregnancy will be. Moreover, all of these studies are based on a highly questionable underlying assumption: that all women who have had three miscarriages share a common difficulty, and therefore have the same odds of overcoming their problem. Unfortunately, none of these studies has investigated what the effect on the outcome of the pregnancy is of a specific problem, such as an incompetent cervix. Until specific problems are isolated and studied, the statistics will have little meaning. The risk of having another miscarriage for the woman who has cervical incompetence is, in fact, quite different from the risk for the woman whose husband is a carrier of a chromosomal abnormality and from that for the woman whose miscarriages were caused by unknown or random factors.

Most physicians recommend that a couple should be medically evaluated if they have had three consecutive miscarriages. However, many couples who have had two miscarriages are unwilling to attempt another pregnancy without knowing whether they may have a treatable problem, and so elect to begin an evaluation after the second miscarriage. It is likely that the physician will be responsive to a couple's preferences in this regard, so one should be sure to make one's wishes known.

In making his assessment your physician will be guided by his knowledge of your unique medical history, the course of each of your pregnancies, pathology reports on fetal tissue, if available, and what he finds when he examines you. A basic evaluation might include a hysterogram (dye is injected through the cervix in order to make the anatomy of the uterine cavity visible), and karyotyping (a study to determine whether either you or your spouse has a structural chromosomal abnormality). A more extensive evaluation might include thyroid function tests, a cervical culture for herpes virus and T-mycoplasma, measurement of serum progesterone, screening for systemic diseases known to predispose a woman to miscarry, and whatever other tests your physician believes may be fruitful.

REPEATED STILLBIRTH AND MULTIPLE LOSSES OF MIXED TYPE

Why some otherwise healthy women seem to be at an increased risk of experiencing repeated pregnancy loss is somewhat of a medical mystery, especially so since the majority of miscarriages and a significant number of stillbirths are caused by random, nonrecurrent factors. Stillbirth is often a result of either natural accidents of labor (such as prolapse of the umbilical cord, or placental abnormalities) or the injudicious conduct of labor or a traumatic delivery.

Less puzzling are those repeated pregnancy losses that occur in women who have either a chronic or recurrent illness or medical condition. There is a known correlation between certain medical problems and an increased rate of pregnancy loss. Among these are diabetes, kidney disease, systemic lupus erythematosis, severe hypertension, and toxemia. For example, the reported mortality rate for fetuses and newborns of diabetic mothers is 5 to 10 percent.

The chance that the fetus of a diabetic mother will be adversely affected is dependent to a considerable degree on how severe the illness, how long the mother has had diabetes, and whether or not she has preexisting kidney or blood-vessel damage as a result of her illness. Similarly, the risk of fetal loss associated with the other conditions listed depends to some extent on how severe the mother's illness is.

If you have had either a stillbirth or a combination of losses, it is critically important that you seek a thorough medical evaluation, preferably with a specialist in high-risk pregnancy. It is possible that you may have a diagnosable disorder, which can be treated, thereby increasing your chance of carrying a pregnancy successfully to term in the future.

Perhaps your problem is not that you don't know why you have lost pregnancies, but that you have to live with knowing that a disease or condition that you have was probably responsible for the reproductive difficulties you have experienced. If this is so, you may find that your ability to deal with both kinds of problems depends on how well you have accepted and accommodated to living with your illness. If you have had to make a major adjustment to living with a disease such as diabetes, you may have already come to terms with many of the issues one has to face when a pregnancy is lost. Having coped with this, you will probably have internal resources you can draw on.

If, on the other hand, you have been only minimally affected by your illness before you lose a pregnancy, you may find that it is particularly difficult to cope simultaneously with the grief that you feel at losing a pregnancy and the grief that you feel at recognizing how strongly your illness may impact on your life. Such is not infrequently the case for the woman with mild to moderate diabetes, for example.

ECTOPIC PREGNANCY: RECURRENCE AND SUBSEQUENT INFERTILITY

The incidence of persistent infertility and recurrent ectopic pregnancy following one ectopic pregnancy is significant. Studies show that 50 percent of women are unable to conceive after having had an ectopic pregnancy. This means that about half the women who have had one ectopic pregnancy will not be able to become pregnant again. Among those who are able to conceive, between 25 and 69 percent will have a subsequent normal intrauterine pregnancy; and between 7 and 12 percent will have another ectopic pregnancy. These statistics indicate that only about one third of the women who have had an ectopic pregnancy can expect to produce a living child.

What does this mean for you? Your chance of being successful may be better or worse than statistics predict, depending on whether or not the problem that caused the ectopic pregnancy involves both tubes or is confined to the affected tube alone; depending on the degree of damage caused by the ectopic pregnancy, on the surgical procedure your phyisican performed, and also depending on other factors that affect your fertility.

If during surgery your physician found that the affected tube was damaged beyond repair, and that your other tube was missing, malformed, or so damaged as to make the possibility of pregnancy unlikely, he will have informed you that your chances of conceiving are nonexistent. If, however, you still have one good tube on the opposite side, he will probably have removed the affected tube. (Leaving a damaged tube in place is considered unwise, because the likelihood that it will obstruct the passage of another ovum, thereby causing another ectopic pregnancy, is significant.) As long as you have one healthy tube remaining, your overall fertility should be adequate to allow conception to occur.

A third possibility is that your affected tube was removed during surgery and that your remaining tube was found to be somewhat damaged. Depending on the extent of the damage, the likelihood that you will be able to conceive an intrauterine pregnancy may be either reasonably good or quite poor. In the latter instance reconstructive tubal surgery may be able to benefit you.

If the condition of your fallopian tube or tubes is not known, your physician will probably want to do a hysterosalpingogram. This involves inserting a special dye into the uterus through the cervix, and then monitoring by X ray its course through the fallopian tube(s) and into the abdominal cavity. By observing whether the dye moves freely through each tube, it is possible to determine whether the passageway is open or whether any obstruction is present. The results of this test will help your physician assess what your chance is of being able to conceive an intrauterine pregnancy, as well as whether or not tubal reconstructive surgery is necessary and feasible.

At the present time, surgery to remove adhesions that obstruct the tubal passageway and surgery to reconstruct a damaged or malformed tube are the only treatments available to women who have obstructed or partially obstructed fallopian tubes. Whether or not these procedures are indicated, and what the chance is that they may be successful, should be assessed by your physician or, if he advises it, by a specialist whom he recommends. Tubal reconstruction is performed by only a small number of specialists; therefore, if it seems that surgical correction may be indicated, you will want to arrange to have a consultation with someone experienced with this procedure.

INFERTILITY

What few people realize is that fetal loss is a form of infertility. Although the term *infertility* is most often used for lack of capability to conceive, it is also used to describe being unable to carry a pregnancy to term. Barbara Eck Menning, R.N., in her classic book *Infertility: A Guide for the Childless Couple*, p. 4, defines infertility as the "inability to conceive a pregnancy after a year or more of regular sexual relations without contraception, *or the inability to carry pregnancies to a live birth.*"

Many couples who have experienced ectopic pregnancy, miscarriage, or stillbirth have a history of having had difficulty conceiving. In the case of ectopic pregnancy, the underlying cause of both infertility and fetal loss is often the same. On the other hand, the relationships among miscarriage, stillbirth, mixed and multiple losses, and infertility are not well understood.

The couple with a history of infertility is apt to feel a double sense of loss when a pregnancy fails, as it was probably long awaited and extremely precious. In addition, as there is a reasonable possibility that a future pregnancy will be hard to conceive, they may experience the lost pregnancy as the loss of their only opportunity to produce a child.

Infertility is painful and demoralizing. Years of trying to conceive, endless medical tests, basal body temperature charts, treatments, and "living by the menstrual cycle" all contribute to the stress that most infertile couples experience. So, too, do the feelings of anger, guilt, shame, sadness, self-doubt, and helplessness. Unfortunately, these painful feelings so familiar to the infertile couple are experienced anew when a pregnancy is lost. Moreover, the couple who has had to grapple with years of uncertainty about whether or not they would ever conceive is faced with a new set of obstacles: if they are able to conceive, will they be able to carry the pregnancy to term successfully? Or, as Lila and Joel put it, "Losing a pregnancy after five years of infertility was like being hit again after we had already been down for the third time. We had no resources left; we felt that all of the fight had been taken out of us; then along came another blow. We were aware of how difficult it was for us to get pregnant, and now it seems that getting pregnant is only half the battle."

An additional deprivation encountered by many couples who have conceived and lost a pregnancy after many years of being infertile is that of a support group. The infertile couple who loses a pregnancy may find that they receive little in the way of either sympathy or support from their infertile peers. When the wife was pregnant, they may have avoided or been avoided by those left behind. This self-protective distancing often continues, even though the pregnancy that began it has since failed.

Although, as a rule, infertile couples who are able to become pregnant are considered more fortunate than those who can't, it is not clear that this is, in fact, always the case. Not only is it extremely painful to lose a pregnancy, but paradoxically, the potential to become pregnant may stand in the way of successfully resolving one's feelings about infertility. The couple with no chance of becoming pregnant is forced to confront this very painful reality. When they have been able to do this, they are able to get on with their lives. The task for the couples whose potential fertility remains unproven is more complicated. For them the rosy red apple is always just out of reach. It is hard to give up when, perhaps on the next try, one may be successful. So repeated attempts continue to be made, often delaying the successful resolution of their dilemma.

SECONDARY INFERTILITY

If you already have one or more children, but are unable to conceive or successfully carry a pregnancy, you are experiencing what physicians refer to as secondary infertility. Secondary infertility can result from any of the same causes as primary infertility. Secondary infertility is always frustrating and baffling. It may be hard to understand why, when everything worked the way it should the first time, you are encountering difficulty conceiving or carrying a pregnancy this time around.

Some couples who have lost a pregnancy find that although they did not have difficulty becoming pregnant the first time, they are not able to become pregnant again. More often than not, the reason is not immediately apparent, and it requires a careful infertility evaluation to diagnose the cause of the difficulty.

The couple who experiences secondary infertility after a pregnancy loss has a doubly heavy burden to bear. Not only do they suffer the loss of the child they were carrying, but in addition, they must contend with a second obstacle in the way of their desire to produce a child. Couples who are in this unfortunate position often find that their grief is quite prolonged. In part this is so because they are mourning not one but two very painful losses. Additionally, because they are unable to produce another child, this means of resolving their loss is not available to them.

Secondary infertility is similar to primary infertility, but in some important ways it is quite different from it. One of the central differences is one of self-definition. Couples who find that they have secondary infertility have not yet defined themselves as infertile. Likewise, since they already have a child or have been able to conceive, the outside world does not define them as infertile, either.

This can make for difficulty. Many couples have found that friends and relatives may either be unaware of their problem, or, if aware, may minimize it. After all, they were able to conceive or produce a child once, weren't they? What is frequently overlooked by outsiders is the couple's intense desire for another child and their pain at not being able to have one.

Because this often is not understood, the secondarily infertile couple often receives very little social support. Comments such as

"Don't worry, dear, you conceived once; of course, you'll be able to do it again" and advice to "get pregnant right away so your children won't be too far apart in age" reflect this attitude. So, too, do remarks intended as offerings of consolation, but often heard as insensitive and hurtful: for example, "Count your blessings; at least you have one" or "How much worse if this had happened to you the first time."

What others may not understand, and what secondarily infertile couples sometimes do not understand themselves, is that although already having a child may ease the pain somewhat, it does not necessarily diminish the longing to have more. Or, put another way, it is at once possible to feel fortunate that you have a child and quite miserable at not being able to have another.

III.

The Experience
of Those Close to You

6. Your Husband and Your Marriage

When a couple suffers a pregnancy loss a man is often faced with many burdens. He must help his wife get through the trauma, physically and emotionally. In addition, he must deal with doctors and tell the bad news to family and friends. Through all this, he must deal with his own emotions of shock, anger, and grief.

The man, too, has lost a child and his hopes and dreams for that child. He probably feels robbed and deeply sad, yet he may find it very difficult to express his feelings. His wife is probably too upset to comfort him, and he feels he must be strong for her and everyone else. Everyone turns to him, but he·has no one to turn to. As a result, he may suppress his emotions and try to act as normal as possible. When asked how he is, he may simply say, "Fine," because he is too embarrassed to discuss his emotions, or fearful he will lose control.

It is likely that his wife is the main recipient of expressions of sympathy and concern. While he realizes that his wife has suffered even more than he has and is in need of support, he may still feel neglected or jealous of the attention she is getting. Alternatively, he may feel glad that no one is probing his feelings, since he prefers to keep them under control.

During the actual loss many men feel afraid for their wives' health. Especially in the case of an ectopic pregnancy, there may be concern that his wife's life is in danger. If he is separated from his wife for any length of time, his fantasies may run wild: what if she doesn't make it? What if they can't stop the bleeding? What if she never comes out of the anesthesia?

Alternatively, he may have been with his wife during labor and delivery, possibly helping with the breathing techniques learned during childbirth classes. It is difficult enough for a man to watch his wife suffer the pains of childbirth when the result is a healthy baby. However, when the baby is dead, the suffering is even harder to bear.

The wife's stay in the hospital, no matter how long it was, is probably a time both would like to forget.

Bob, whose wife, Pat, stayed in the postpartum ward for three days following a stillbirth, describes his reaction to his wife's hospital stay: "The days when Pat was in the hospital were extremely hard on me. I spent as much time as I could at her bedside. I was the only one she wanted to see and I wanted to be with her. I hated watching the pain she was in and seeing her drugged. She was so upset, she cried almost constantly. I didn't know what to say to make her feel better. It seemed as if there were no words, so I held her a lot and told her how much I loved her and that we'd try again as soon as we could. I listened over and over again as she recounted the delivery and poured out her feelings. It nearly broke my heart to see her that way. At night I went home and cried myself to sleep."

If the pregnancy terminated in a stillbirth, hospital personnel probably consulted with the father about what arrangements to make for the baby's body and whether a funeral was desired. Some men make the decision themselves, preferring not to submit their wives to additional stress. Others consult with their wives to find out their preferences and let them participate in the decision if they want to.

Regardless of the way it is handled, the question of arrangements for the body of a stillborn child is probably one of the most unpleasant tasks a man has to face.

RETURNING HOME

The husband probably feels relieved and glad when his wife is discharged and able to return to the privacy of their home. At the same time, he may dread facing the enormity of their loss. He may have been able to keep up a front in the hospital, but at home he is fearful of being overwhelmed with his emotions. He worries about the effect his emotions will have on his devastated wife.

In addition, he may be unprepared for the intensity of his wife's reaction to their loss. She is exhausted, in pain, depressed, irritable, and angry, unceasingly, it seems. She may cry a great deal and snap at him for no reason. It seems as if she is crying hysterically as he leaves for work in the morning; she is still in tears when he calls during the day to check on her; and the tears are still flowing when he comes home.

If she does not get over her grief, he may find that he craves some escape. It surprises him to find that he is tempted to get away, to work late, to take overnight business trips — anything to get a break. He knows he's a bastard for wanting to escape, but he can't stand it anymore. The fact that his wife can't escape, but he can, makes him feel all the more guilty for wanting to.

His efforts to cheer up his wife fail. He can't even get her to smile. He attempts to change the subject, but she keeps talking about the whole ordeal over and over again in explicit detail. He is sick of hearing about it and wishes she could put this behind her and go on with her life.

Her intense feelings of loss and sadness continue past the time he feels they should. Weeks or months have passed and she doesn't seem to be getting any better. He starts to wonder if there is something wrong with her — maybe she is neurotic; possibly she should see a psychiatrist or be hospitalized. During this period a man may be confused by his conflicting feelings toward his wife. On the one hand, he sympathizes with her pain and knows how important the baby was to her. On the other hand, he may be irritable with her and lack patience for her continuing grief.

BELATED REACTION

A number of couples reported that the man experienced a belated reaction to the pregnancy loss. As much as several months afterward, the husband may feel intense emotions not unlike what his wife felt immediately after the trauma. Initially he may have suppressed his emotions as he comforted his wife. As time passes and she begins to recover, he may find that his emotions surface and must be dealt with. All through the crisis, he had been able to carry on as usual at work and at home. Now he may be irritable, angry, jealous of couples with children, fearful of death, and depressed. He may never have experienced such strong emotions and may have difficulty expressing them. Because some weeks or months have passed since the loss, he may not even associate these feelings with the trauma.

Many males have been discouraged from showing their feelings. In this situation, however, it helps to let feelings emerge, to feel the pain, to cry. To recover fully, he too must pass through the various stages of mourning. (See chapter 1 for fuller discussion of grieving.)

THE MARITAL RELATIONSHIP

The loss of a pregnancy inevitably causes stress to each marital partner. Often the marital relationship is strained as well. However, despite the fact that the going may have been rough for a while, many couples have felt that sharing their grief over their lost pregnancy has brought them closer together. Sometimes we show a part of ourselves in times of crisis that we keep hidden at other times. Whatever the hidden aspect, whether it was an ability to cope, sensitivity, or optimism, there may be pleasure in discovering each other and in knowing each other more fully.

Some couples have found that they were strengthened as individuals and as a partnership by being able to comfort each other and by understanding what the other person was going through. To share feelings and to make it through together can lay the foundation for the development of a more trusting and intimate relationship. There is also satisfaction to be gained from feeling that one was faced with something hard, and that together the pair found a way to handle it.

One woman described the bond between herself and her husband following the loss of their pregnancy at eight months: "We went through it together, every step of the way: the pain, the hope, the anger, the feelings of isolation, and the decisions at each step. I couldn't imagine not having him to share it with. We cried together and got angry together. Our relationship grew stronger as he and I together faced all the babies and pregnant ladies in the grocery store."

Another woman, Sarah, spoke of the effect of her stillbirth on her relationship with her husband, John. "We became closer than ever. John was not ashamed to cry in my arms, nor I in his. The grief would not hit us at the same time during the months that followed, but we were always sensitive and supportive when it did hit. My husband was very upset, and during this time, for the first time ever, I saw him cry. I know he was very hurt. We both wanted the baby desperately. John still has a special spot on his jogging trail on the top of a mountain, where he stops to think about her."

Sarah's words reflect the thoughts of many women. Her husband's reaction to the loss helped her become aware of the depth of his love and devotion. Coming at a time of great vulnerability, this reassurance was especially welcome.

She took comfort in the fact that John grieved over the loss and she felt better knowing that he, too, was hurt and had yearned to have a child. She felt optimistic that she and he would be parents someday, either by giving birth or adopting. Knowing that John wanted a family as much as she did helped Sarah cope with her grief and look toward the future.

PULLING APART

Pregnancy loss can strain even the best of relationships. Couples who have relatively stable and longstanding relationships may find themselves arguing, feeling misunderstood, resenting one another, or withdrawing completely.

If this is your experience, you may find this breakdown of communication distressing. After all, you are in the middle of a crisis, and feeling close to your spouse is more important than ever. Friction between you only adds to your tremendous emotional burden. It is not uncommon to feel as if everything were going wrong all at once. First, you lost your baby, now you feel at times as if you are losing your husband, and maybe your mind. Try to remember that both of you are going through a crisis and, given the complex nature of what you have been through, there is much room for communication to break down.

To understand why problems so frequently arise, it is important to realize that the psychological experience of losing a pregnancy is most likely very different for the man and for the woman. Most women form an emotional attachment to their future child early in the pregnancy, while most men feel little or no attachment until late in the pregnancy, or form an attachment only after the child is born. This is because the woman experiences pregnancy more directly — she senses the early signs and symptoms and later feels the baby move inside her. Her husband can experience the pregnancy only through his wife's words and observations. A woman who suffered two miscarriages commented: "A man doesn't sense the physical bonding a mother does. I don't think my husband related to the fetuses as babies — real persons — as I did. He did not have the physical pain, humiliation, or hormonal ups and downs that I did. He surely wasn't happy about these miscarriages, but he did not experience the losses as strongly or significantly as I did."

It follows, then, that because each parent has a different attachment, each will have a different response to the loss of a child early in pregnancy. The mother mourns the loss as she would the loss of a beloved person. The father, who in all likelihood has not yet formed as strong an attachment to the child, feels saddened by the death, but probably does not mourn as though he were grieving for a person.

"My husband was understanding but couldn't know what this did to my whole sense of myself," said Karen following her miscarriage. "After months of my moping and lack of interest, he wondered if I wasn't prolonging things and overreacting. I started resenting him for having escaped the full emotional burden of the loss. It was a difficult time for us. I think it is impossible for a man to understand miscarriage on anything but an intellectual level."

When partners do not understand that each of them has formed a different kind of attachment to their future child, they are likely to be confused and angered by their spouses' responses to the loss. The husband may feel that his wife is overreacting and she may be furious with her husband for being less affected than she is by the loss.

Donna describes her experience: "In a moment of tenseness, when we were both exhausted, he finally confronted me with his feeling that by this time I should have had more perspective. His insensitivity confirmed my estrangement from him. I also felt foolish at not having realized before that we were so different."

The duration of the pregnancy may partly determine how the husband reacts to the loss: the longer the pregnancy, the more attached he is likely to feel to the baby. In the case of ectopic pregnancy, the husband may not have known of the pregnancy before it was discovered. Even if he did know, his wife was probably no more than two months along. Similarly, when miscarriage occurs early in pregnancy, the husband has had little or no time to get used to the idea of having a baby or to become emotionally invested in the pregnancy. Carol, who miscarried at four and a half months, remarked: "I was totally disappointed in my husband at the time. As far as he was concerned, there really was no pregnancy. He could not experience the grief that I was going through. He was very sympathetic to my fears but not to my grief. I often said to him that I wished that I had broken an arm or a leg so that he could see my wound and understand."

The man is apt to be most affected when the loss occurs late in pregnancy or when a child is stillborn. As many months have passed, he, too, has experienced fantasies of the expected baby. Chances are he has put his hand on his wife's abdomen to feel the baby kick or has heard its heart beat. When his future child has become a reality to him; he is likely to mourn its loss in much the same way as his wife does.

RECOGNIZING THAT EACH PERSON MUST MOURN IN HIS OWN WAY AND IN HIS OWN TIME

When couples are able to share their feelings, they are better able to resolve their misunderstandings, especially when one partner is mistaken about the other's emotional state. Judy told us: "My husband was a bulwark of strength throughout everything. With my first miscarriage my husband was told by my mother to be strong for my sake. I found this out much later. This caused him to cover up his grief. I attributed his normalcy to lack of caring. Communication between us broke down almost entirely. It took months for him to admit that he was in pain just like me. We learned from our past experience and grieved together after our second miscarriage."

Patty reports a similar experience after her ectopic pregnancy.

"He was more upset than I realized as he tried to hide his feelings. I felt bitter and angry at the world that I had lost a baby and then had to go through the discomfort of surgery, too. Not until several months after the ectopic pregnancy were my husband and I finally able to share our feelings. We cried together and then felt much better. I think each of us tried to put up a front for the other. My husband's grief was as deep as mine, but I didn't know it at first. There was a lot of tension during the several months when I felt he wasn't disturbed much at all. Since we finally had it out and I learned his feelings, everything has been fine."

Some women viewed their husbands' reactions to the loss as typical of their way of coping with crisis. Their husbands' style was to grieve for a short time, get over it quickly, and go on with life. These men often failed to understand that their wives needed more time than they did to get over the death.

"My husband's grief was equal to mine, but he resolved it sooner," Joyce said. "He cried a lot the first day but composed himself a lot more quickly than I did. He generally accepts things better than I do. He doesn't dwell on something. He prefers to accept and set things aside — to go on in a positive fashion. He thought my feelings should have been handled and let go sooner than they were. He viewed my grieving as unnecessary and counterproductive. He kept telling me it was in the past and I should go on with my life."

Another woman, Sandy, said of her husband: "He was unhappy to lose the baby but felt there was no point in mourning what could not be changed. He was more upset for me than for himself. Ultimately, he was disturbed by the fact that I could not get over my grief. He felt badly for me, yet he simply did not understand me."

Hurt feelings and fears that your husband does not share your grief are not easy to cope with. Try to give your partner the benefit of the doubt. It is likely that he is suffering, too. Put yourself in his place and try to imagine how you would react. In addition, try not to assume anything. Before interpreting your spouse's behavior, ask him what it means. You may save yourself a lot of pain and grief.

Communicate your feelings to each other. What you're going

through is real and deserves to be shared. This should help you to grow as individuals and as a couple.

"I tried to push my husband away at first," said Lynn. "I felt that losing him would be just punishment for someone like me who couldn't even perform a normal biological function. I finally realized that losing him would be worse than losing the baby. Our marriage has been loving, strong, and happy ever since."

Try to resist the temptation to withdraw from your spouse. You need one another now. If you notice that your partner is emotionally isolated, make a special effort to open lines of communication.

One woman commented: "Since we weren't able to talk, my husband took a position where he traveled a lot, and wasn't home very often. This led to more misunderstanding and almost to the breakup of our marriage. We couldn't help each other work through our loss, so we felt sad and alone."

Another said: "I couldn't talk to my husband about feelings that made sense to him. I cried a lot, sat and didn't talk for an hour at a time. It frustrated him. Neither of us knew how to cope."

SOURCES OF MARITAL TROUBLE

Many spouses experience difficulty understanding each other's feelings after a pregnancy loss. It is often difficult for the husband to comprehend the intensity of his wife's pain, since he did not share her physical experience of the pregnancy or her strong emotional attachment to it. Similarly, it may be difficult for the wife to appreciate her husband's pain. If he is not open about his feelings or if she is so depleted by her own physical and emotional anguish that she is unable to be aware of anything else, she may fail to recognize that he too is grieving.

Difficulties may also arise if a partner openly or secretly blames the other for doing or not doing something that may have affected the outcome of the pregnancy: for example, participating in an activity such as sports, work, or travel. Sometimes one partner may blame the other for having had ambivalent feelings early in the pregnancy, as in the following situation. "The pregnancy was not a loss to him. It didn't represent a baby as it did to me," said a woman who miscarried at almost four months. "I developed a great deal of resentment for what I felt was his lack of grief and never hesitated to say, 'Well, you never wanted that baby anyway.' "

One spouse may project his or her own ambivalence onto the other spouse and then feel angry with him or her for having those feelings. If you find you are blaming your spouse for causing the loss, stop and think. Maybe your need to blame comes from your own anger, guilt, or need to find a reason. Remember, it is very unusual for pregnancy loss to be caused by something anyone did. Similarly, if your partner blames you for causing the loss, help him or her see that it was no one's fault. It may be helpful for both partners to visit their doctor together to hear his explanation; any questions about possible causes can be resolved at that time.

It is not uncommon for one or both partners to fear that they will be abandoned by a disappointed or angry spouse. Some couples "act out" these fears by testing or provoking each other. In the following case, the wife acted on a mistaken assumption. After her second miscarriage, Miriam felt convinced that her husband of five years would surely want to leave her to marry a woman who could have children. She began to withdraw and to become increasingly unavailable to him to minimize the hurt she would feel when he actually left. Although he was patient at first, Carl eventually found himself increasingly irritated with Miriam's withdrawal. During a major confrontation between them, Carl told Miriam that he felt emotionally abandoned by her, and she was able to tell him of her fear that he would leave her. Had this not been so, Miriam might have continued to behave in such a way as to bring about the reaction from Carl that she feared most.

Another difficulty sometimes encountered by couples who have lost a baby is that either partner, or sometimes both partners, may experience a short-lived or longer-lasting decrease in sexual desire. This may be the result of an underlying depression, or it may be related to anxiety, feelings of inadequacy, fear of conceiving another pregnancy, or pressure to conceive again. One or both partners may feel that sex has become a chore. "Sex wasn't fun anymore" is the way one woman expressed it. The anger, fear, or anxiety thus engendered may further compound already present problems.

Try not to panic about your sexual difficulties. Most likely, they are a reaction to stressful circumstances and will improve as time passes and as you and your partner begin to feel better.

Counseling should be considered if after several months have passed either or both of you continue to feel emotionally estranged, angry, depressed, or unable to function. The loss of your pregnancy may be the first crisis you have faced together, and you may need help in dealing with it. Counseling can help you define your problems and cope with them more effectively.

One Man's Story

My wife, Alaina, gave birth to our daughter by cesarean section; I was present at the delivery. I was as unprepared initially for the stillbirth as the doctors were. Our baby had four congenital heart defects, which were undetected during pregnancy (through no fault of our obstetrician) due to the fact that while the baby was in the womb, Alaina's body supplied the necessary biological functions to keep the baby alive, masking the heart deficiencies. During delivery, when she was subjected to stress and when Alaina's life-support systems were removed, our daughter was not able to survive on her own. The thought that maybe something could be wrong with our baby had occurred to Alaina and me but, like many parents-to-be, we had given it little serious thought.

Within the space of a few short hours we experienced the thrill and excitement of expecting an apparently perfect child, and then the blackest despair when we discovered that our baby had died.

When the doctors quietly told me that our baby was dead, it didn't matter to me that they were in tears or that the nurses were obviously deeply affected. Alaina and I felt alone, deserted by life. We didn't want to talk with anyone about what had happened, because we felt so alone and helpless. We found ourselves searching for answers, for solutions to the emotional turmoil we were experiencing. It was a very personal grief, which continued for days and weeks afterward.

Where could we turn for help? Friends? Our parents? Doctors, nurses?

Immediately after the doctors gave us the bad news, I phoned my father and Alaina's parents with the news. They would then tell others in our immediate families, as I was too upset to do so. Sometimes it is hard enough for a person to cope with his own emotions, much less those of others.

Alaina and I felt that it was important that an autopsy be performed, since we hoped to learn what had caused our baby to die and thus, if possible, to prevent such occurrences in the future. Our consent was required, and I had to sign a form giving the doctors permission. I felt almost as if I had received a physical blow as I signed my name to that piece of paper.

Immediately after our daugher's death Alaina and I wanted to be alone; we felt too emotionally drained to deal with others just then.

I remained with Alaina in the hospital for two days, in the same room, sleeping in a recliner chair the nurses had thoughtfully provided; they realized what Alaina and I were going through and were magnificent in their understanding and generous with their help. The maternity ward personnel were very aware of life and death and the impact of both on the parents. Alaina and I needed each other very much, and this time was quite important for us. Little was said, but the fact that we were together was a comfort. I ignored my job and outside responsibilities. I felt that my first responsibility was to Alaina; everything else was secondary. I stayed with her constantly, attending to her needs, simply being there to help if she needed me.

After the first heartbreaking hours passed, the relatives had been notified, the various official forms had been signed, and other details completed, I was in a state of physical and mental exhaustion. I had not slept more than three hours at a stretch in three days. Whenever I went home to rest after those initial days, I always returned as quickly as possible; I felt very uncomfortable when I was not with my wife.

When I was home, our son, Christopher and I were together constantly. After telling him what had happened, I answered his questions about his baby sister and about why she wouldn't be coming home to her new room that he had helped us decorate. I was amazed at the wealth of understanding Christopher displayed; he was hurt, sad, and confused, but he always told me: "I love you, Daddy, and I won't go away." He wasn't very old at the time, just past three, but he grasped what had taken place and, with the innocence of the young, helped his daddy to cope with it. He has always been a special boy, and is even more so now.

I assumed much of the burden of worldly affairs; I had to make various arrangements, and I had to act as a buffer between Alaina and the world in gen-

eral. There were many things that had to be dealt with, important issues that could not wait, that had to be faced. For instance, I had to decide who visited, the length of time visitors remained, and the emotional and physical impact these visits might have on Alaina.

Although people mean well, care for you, and want to help, visits can be tiring. We found that both of us were gladdened at the display of concern but at the same time exhausted by it. In general, we tried to keep visits short.

After three days Alaina was moved from the maternity section to the surgery recovery floor. Because she had had a cesarean section, the time she spent in the hospital was longer than for a normal delivery. The psychological implications of this move, we found, were enormous and difficult. Her removal from the ward concerned with new life and happiness to another dedicated to recovery from physical trauma caused us both pain; the last link between us and our baby had been severed.

We found that the nurses on the surgery ward didn't know what had happened to us. At least four nurses asked either Alaina or me how our new baby was doing. It became annoying the second, third, and fourth times I had to explain that our daughter had died.

Alaina was released from the hospital after nearly five days, and we finally found ourselves at home. Before she came home, I did whatever household chores were necessary and had everything ready for her return; it didn't seem right to have her come home to anything other than a clean house.

Just as we had started to recover, reality struck again; the baby's burial had to be arranged. Earlier, while we were still at the hospital, I had made arrangements with our local mortuary to transport the body to their facilities for cremation. One of the worst experiences I had was going to the mortuary to obtain our daughter's ashes. I held them in my hands; a small wrapped box of ashes was all that remained of our hopes and dreams.

When the plot and headstone were ready, my father kindly took the ashes to the cemetery, had them buried and the headstone installed. The ashes were interred with my grandfather and grandmother in our family plot in a quiet, tree-shaded cemetery in a small rural town where my father and his family grew up.

After this was done Alaina and I had to make the decision as to whether we wanted to have a funeral service or not. We did not have a service. We felt that our baby was too new to the world for others to feel as strongly about her as we did. We also felt that a funeral service would only compound the grief we already felt. Outside pressures (societal, family, religious, and so on) were strong, but I made it known to everyone who mattered that our mutual decision was not to have a formal service. Alaina and I would take care of it in our own way.

Soon after our arrival home, doctor bills, hospital bills, and other reminders began to arrive. These were a continual reminder of what had taken place. The past kept intruding into the present: this went on for months, especially when we began receiving advertisements for various new-parent and new-baby magazines.

Friends and family sometimes offered their opinions, thoughts, and suggestions about what we should be doing, both for the moment and in the future. The flow of comments and advice began about a week after we had lost the baby. The absolutely worst things that were said to us were "Well, it just wasn't meant to be." Or: "It's God's will." Or: "You and your wife are being tested." Or: "Forget about having children and just proceed as if nothing happened. Do what you want to do and forget about kids."

We listened politely, nodded our heads, and then ignored, or tried to ignore, what had been said. We knew we would decide what was right for us. However, after hearing the same "suggestions" over and over again for weeks, I found it increasingly difficult to remain silent. Once, I even blew up at an acquaintance who gave me the "You're being tested" line.

I myself was more than a little bitter about what had happened. If what happened to us was a "test," then it was a grotesque and cruel test that was totally unnecessary. I couldn't comprehend then, and I don't now, any reason for what happened to our baby and our family. We had done everything correctly, had not endangered the unborn child in any fashion, and had every reason to expect the delivery of a perfectly healthy and normal child. I am still upset that our child was taken from us; it was not fair. It was cruel. This reaction is, I feel, perfectly justified and normal; I have no guilt about feeling as I do, and I expect others to respect my feelings.

After I had been back at work for two weeks I found that I was dreading going to the office. In my business, I deal with the public; this meant that I had to explain two or three times a day that our baby had died. Some well-meaning person would ask how our new little one was getting along, and I then had to go over it all again.

Our depression and unease continued for months; at first, we felt down much of the time. As the days passed, however, our outlook gradually improved, and emotional lows occurred less frequently. Still, grief continued to strike periodically for weeks and months afterward. We weren't prepared for this, and it was rough.

Often I struggled with my emotions and my memories of all that had happened. I couldn't keep all of the emotional by-products bottled up inside; I am thankful to have some close friends with whom I was able to discuss what I was feeling. I found that it was good to be able to talk to someone outside the immediate family at times. Mostly, it was helpful to talk with Alaina. I found that sharing our feelings with each other brought us closer together than we had ever been. We had planned together for our child, prepared ourselves for the new addition, dealt with the pregnancy for nine months, attended the birth, and coped with the death together, Alaina and I.

And yet . . . our baby is gone.

7. Children, Family, and Friends

Besides your spouse, the other members of your immediate family affected by your pregnancy loss are your children. One dilemma of parenthood is introducing and handling the topic of death. What do you tell your child? How many details? How can it be described so that he or she understands and is not frightened? At what age are children aware of death? All of these same questions and concerns arise when a pregnancy is lost.

Since pregnancy loss and death are uncomfortable topics, there is a tendency to want to avoid them as much as possible. We convince ourselves that a grandparent's death can be explained by saying he went away on a long trip. We want to spare our children exposure to sadness and the trauma of a death in the family. After an early pregnancy loss, we tell ourselves that a young child couldn't know that anything unusual happened. When he, too, was prepared for a baby brother or sister, we try to soften the message, possibly creating confusion.

But when we do not deal with death openly and sensitively, our children sense that this is a topic that can't be talked about. Although our intention is to protect them from a painful and uncomfortable issue, unfortunately we teach them that death is something to fear, something so bad that it can't even be discussed. Children will also remain silent about the loss of a pregnancy if they think that the subject is taboo. Not knowing what actually happened, they may create fantasies that are often more frightening to them than the real tragedy. (Children frequently deal with the unknown by creating a fantasy to explain things.) Thus, wrapping the loss in silence and secrecy can lead to worse fears than the reality would.

Besides, such secrecy is usually unsuccessful, because children tend to be keenly aware of everything that goes on in the family: they sense sadness, tension, and subtle changes in their parents' behavior. They also have a way of overhearing conversations, of being awake when we are sure they are asleep, and of seeing and hearing more than we are willing to acknowledge. Moreover, most children are able to read the subtle cues (through body language, for instance) that indicate what your real feelings are, even if you try to hide them.

"When I came home from the hospital, my son would sit next to me and hold my hand," one mother said. "It was sweet and comforting. He didn't even know about the miscarriage, but he seemed to sense that something was wrong."

How your child will experience the loss of your pregnancy is determined by many factors: his age, his personality, his past experiences with death, his awareness of your pregnancy, what he witnessed of the loss, how you reacted to the loss, and how you responded to him during this time.

Initially, most children are puzzled and confused. They want to know what happened, why it happened and how. In answering these questions, it is important to remember that your child's understanding is limited by his current level of development. He may not be able to comprehend what you tell him about the death of a potential sibling, but the discussion of it with him will set a pattern of openness and sharing.

In preschool children, several factors may account for confusion or fear about death. The young child has difficulty grasping the finality of death, for one thing. Also, young children often think of themselves as the center of their own world and therefore responsible for everything that happens in it. Further, they have a strong belief in magic. If the child is angry with you, he or she may wish for you to disappear or die. After learning of an expected new child, he or she could feel threatened or jealous and wish the baby would disappear or die. Consequently, if the baby dies, the child may feel that his or her wish caused the baby's death. She or he needs to be assured that this was not so. It is important she or he knows that these wishes did not hurt either you or the baby. If the child believes that he or she caused the baby's death, he or she might come to feel that aggressive wishes could cause other tragedies and may become fearful of the power of his or her own thoughts.

The best way to avoid such fears is to supply your child, even if he or she is quite young, with a clear, simple explanation, appropriate to the child's age, that will give him or her a real way of understanding what happened. For example, one might tell a very young child: "The baby was born when it was too small to live, so we are not going to have a new baby." It is not necessary, or even desirable, to give children all the details. Tell them just enough to make the issue comprehensible, then let them take the lead in asking you what they want to know.

SUGGESTIONS FOR DEALING WITH YOUR CHILD

The following is a model for dealing with your child's thoughts and feelings about the loss. It is based on suggestions discussed by Carol Hardgrove and Louise Warrick in "How Shall We Tell the Children?"

Offer a simple, clear explanation in language and concepts understandable to a child of his or her age. For example, here is what one couple said about telling their four-year-old: "We told her that it was not a baby but a seed for a baby. Later, we told her not all seeds grow. She had this concept from growing a garden."

Use correct words, such as *death* and *died,* rather than euphemisms. Describing death as a long sleep, for instance, may bewilder children and even cause them to fear sleep. Such a comparison and other distortions of death should be avoided, for they may bring more problems in the long run.

Elicit your child's thoughts and feelings. This is best done by asking questions such as "Have you been thinking about the baby a lot?"

If your child does not ask questions spontaneously, take the initiative and seek his or her own explanations of how babies develop, how they are born, and what he thinks happened to the baby you were carrying. This gives you important cues as to what information, corrections, and explanations are needed.

Answer questions when you are asked. One useful way of dealing with them is first to ask your child the same question you have just been asked. For example, when your child asks you what happened to the baby, you can respond: "What do *you* think happened?" In this way, children can express their concepts and feelings while providing you feedback to help you deal with them.

If you use books to explain, you should be familiar with the content before introducing them to your child; then you can discuss the material with her or him. Simply handing the child a book and suggesting he or she read it indicates that you are uncomfortable with the subject and implies that birth and death cannot be spoken of. Several books are listed in the bibliography.

If your child is familiar with religious beliefs, death can be discussed in a religious way, such as that the soul went to heaven or the baby is an angel now. It is best to avoid an expression such as "God took the baby" lest the child become afraid of being taken next.

Continue to raise the matter of the baby's death for months afterward. Also make it easy for your child to raise questions or talk about what happened. Parents should realize that the loss of a pregnancy, though once explained, may dwell in children's thoughts and come up again. Children usually need time to ponder, to understand. Questions will arise weeks or months later, either because something new has happened in their world or because they have reached a new developmental level that makes certain new concepts possible.

Convey to children that there is nothing that cannot be talked about, no question that cannot be asked. However, parents do not need to pretend that they have all of the answers. It is all right to say, "I don't know why that happened."

Respect children's defenses. They do not need, nor will they profit from, an overdose of reality. It is not necessary or advisable for children to accept and assimilate everything all at once. Give them time.

Be expressive of your own feelings of sadness and don't hide them from your child. This will allow him or her to express feelings of sadness without being in a position of needing to protect you from his or her feelings.

CHILDREN'S REACTIONS

Each child reacts to his mother's losing a baby uniquely. Even children who have been carefully prepared often behave in unexpected ways. Since this is a new experience for you and your child, there is a large element of uncertainty that makes it difficult to anticipate exactly what the effect will be.

In understanding your child's reaction, you should keep in mind that you may know very little about how he or she experienced the loss or about what he or she believes happened. Very young children may be unable to verbalize their thoughts about it. If they feel guilty or responsible, if they feel that somehow they killed the baby or that you did, or if they feel disappointed or deprived, their reactions are apt to reflect this.

"Our four-year-old was disappointed and frustrated when we told her," one mother said. "She asked, 'Is it because you didn't take care of it?' 'No,' I replied, 'I did everything I could. It just wasn't the right seed.' She said angrily, 'Well you should have gotten a book that told you the right way to take care of it.' "

In addition, your child's reactions will be less baffling to you if you remember that children grieve differently from adults. Some psychiatrists think that children are incapable of true mourning until adolescence. Before this time, they do not have the ability really to understand death or to cope with it by internalizing the loss. If you don't understand this, your child's apparent lack of concern or newly acquired behavioral problems may be confusing. Children often express feelings of grief in their actions rather than in words. Some children may appear whiny and difficult, others may be aggressive or destructive; still others may be angry, withdrawn, or clinging. Be on the lookout for unusual behavior, which may be an indication that your child is struggling with painful feelings or frightening or disturbing thoughts or fantasies.

A mother who miscarried said: "Our daughter seemed fine all along and then one day she tried to push the fish tank over. I was shocked, as she was always so perfectly behaved. After much discussion, she was able to tell me that she thought that if the baby died inside of me, I would die, too. I assured her that this was not so. She wanted to know how the baby would get out, or if it would just stay inside me. I explained fully and factually. After that, she had no more fears or behavior problems and was fine."

Following is a small sample of the ways in which some children have reacted to the death of a potential sister or brother.

"Our four-year-old's grief was not as obvious as ours after the stillbirth. He cried when we told him of her death. I noticed that his finger paintings became very dark, colorless, and shapeless for a couple of months. He still talks about her and wishes that she was here to play with him."

"Our two-year-old was angry, sad, and disappointed. She reflected our sadness. A few months later our three-year-old suddenly became clingy."

A third mother remarked: "After my ectopic, my two-and-a-half-year-old son was very upset about my being in the hospital and away from him. It took him a number of months to accept having a babysitter after that."

It is important for parents to read behavioral signs that indicate distress. If troubling behavior is present, you should try to determine what may be bothering your child. If the child is verbal, ask him or her what he is worried about, or suggest areas of concern that you think might be disturbing him. If the child can't express himself verbally, situation role-playing may be useful. Similarly, parents can use dolls or storytelling to help their children talk about events that occurred in the life of the doll or fictional character, which mirror events in the child's own life. For example, you could start a game by saying, "When mother doll went to the hospital . . ."

Some parents have found that the family physician or the child's pediatrician may be willing either to offer advice on how to deal with the child's concerns or to deal directly with the child. If this latter situation occurs, it is critical that you be present when the doctor speaks with your child.

Occasionally, a child may have a significantly disturbed reaction to losing a potential sibling. Any intense reaction that does not seem to diminish spontaneously over time is a cause for concern and should be discussed with your pediatrician. He or she may be able to offer you valuable suggestions for helping your child. He will also be able to assess whether counseling may be useful in helping your child deal with his feelings.

ANTICIPATING THE CHILD'S NEEDS

The parent who recognizes that his child may well be affected when a potential sibling is lost is in a position to anticipate his very special needs during this difficult time. First, you should be aware that the issue of death is frightening to almost all children. Like adults, they may feel an increased sense of personal vulnerability when someone close to them dies. "After my stillbirth," Alice said, "my three-and-a-half-year-old daughter asked me endless questions about dying. She became fearful of death since she knew it would mean that she'd never see us again."

One way to diminish your child's feelings of vulnerability is to point out to him or her that he is not in danger: a simple statement such as "The baby was very small and not strong enough to live yet; not like you, you're a big, strong, and healthy child." This should help him or her to feel safer. Physical closeness with children is another way of telling them that they are not alone, that they are loved and that you won't let anything bad happen to them.

It is important to convey the message that it is all right to feel sad or frightened, to cry, to wonder, or to express feelings of anger or relief. Your acceptance of the child's feelings is a way of communicating your acceptance of her or him. Moreover, it lets your child know that such feelings are appropriate when someone important has been lost. In this way your child learns that grieving is normal.

Possibly, your child might experience your preoccupation with a baby who has died as a rejection of him or her, or as a message that he or she was lacking in some way: why else would you be so upset? Reassurance that the child is important, special, and loved often goes a long way toward alleviating these feelings. Similarly, the child may need reassurance that he or she has not lost his or her special place in the family. Verbal reassurance, physical closeness, and special time spent together are all ways of letting the child know that she or he is important to you.

Resist withdrawing into depression. Try not to leave your child's care to someone else or to minister to external needs while neglecting a more intimate relationship with him or her. Predictably, you are feeling exhausted, preoccupied, and depleted. You're not sure how much you have to give anyone. Nevertheless, make the effort to stay in close contact with your child during this stressful time. This will afford him maximum comfort and security and will also help keep you in communication. In addition, the comfort you derive both from seeing your child through this family crisis and from the closeness that you have created can be wonderfully healing for you as well.

FAMILY AND FRIENDS

You will find that in addition to coping with your own feelings and those of members of your immediate family, you will be affected by the reactions of others, most commonly other family members and friends, to your loss. Not only will you be aware of their reactions to you, you will be mindful of your responses to them.

The loss of your baby probably has had an effect on the people around you. What your friends and family have in common is that they are likely to feel sad that your pregnancy ended as disastrously as it did. However, their personal reactions to your loss may vary tremendously, as does their capacity to communicate their feelings to you.

You may be especially grateful to some people for doing and saying all the "right" things and you may feel angry toward others for what they said or didn't say. Certain people "will never be forgotten" for their emotional support while others "will never be forgiven" for their lack of it.

Former patterns of communication with friends and family will probably continue during this time of crisis. If certain people have been supportive in the past, chances are you can depend on them now. Usually, there are a few people in your life whom you call first whenever something significant happens. They will probably be the first over to see you; caring for you as they do, they will want to be with you and share your grief. You will, no doubt, find that talking things over with people who care about you really helps.

REACTIONS TO YOUR LOSS

While generally the nature of your relationships will continue unchanged during your trauma, you may be in for some surprises, both pleasant and unpleasant. Individual friends and family members may not be totally predictable in their reactions to your loss. Similarly, you may have some unexpected responses to others that may confuse you. Let us try to understand these unforeseen reactions and put them in perspective.

You may be pleasantly surprised to get a sympathetic call or note from a person you did not consider a close friend or relative — one whom you haven't spoken to in months, or even seen in years — who has heard about your loss through the grapevine. Such communication is welcome, since it is always nice to know there are people who understand your misfortune. This contact may even lead to a close friendship.

Many couples have found that after a pregnancy has been lost, friends, relatives, and acquaintances who have experienced similar losses are apt to share their own experiences with them. Often one learns of a friend's or relative's lost pregnancy only after having a loss yourself. Most people have found that being able to talk to other people who have also lost a pregnancy is a tremendous help to them. People who have themselves been through something similar will have a good understanding of what you are feeling. In addition, they will probably be able to give you invaluable advice and support. Beverly passed along this letter written by her mother-in-law, Isabel, after Beverly and her husband lost their second baby. Isabel had suffered both a stillbirth and an ectopic pregnancy before her son, Bob, was born. The couple found the letter a great source of comfort and encouragement. Isabel, more than anyone, knew the anguish they felt and they turned to her constantly for support; she was always consoling.

Dear Children,
    Your phone call tonight informing me of the loss of your baby moved me so deeply that I must write. Beverly, dear, when you said, "It looks as if you won't be a grandmother," I'm so sorry. I must say that the thought hadn't occurred to me. All I could feel at the time was how desperately distressed you both must be.
    Having lost two babies before you were born, Bob, I know the feeling of utter loss, the emptiness, the enormous disappointment you both must be experiencing now.
    I mourn with you. My only words of comfort are that fortunately

you are both young and well. Let us hope brighter times will come in the not too far future.

I love you both,
MOTHER

What may surprise and upset you will be the seeming insensitivity and lack of concern from people you thought cared about you. You may feel hurt and let down. You are probably confused by their inability to provide the support you need. You wonder, "Why doesn't she call me? Why do they pretend nothing has happened? Why do they tell me to just forget it and go on with my life?"

It is common to encounter parents and friends who refuse to talk about the loss at all or who want to forget about the whole thing. Pregnancy loss is a time when people learn things about those close to them that may not be very pleasant to face — that some parents are self-centered, concerned with their own needs and unable to give to their grown children, for instance. With effort and attempts to communicate, some of these negative reactions might change. However, some attitudes may never change, and one must then accept this.

One woman told of her family's reaction at the time of her ectopic pregnancy: "They didn't know what to say, so they said nothing. Their silence was very painful to me and caused me ill feelings that will never heal. I wanted them to acknowledge our pain and they ignored it. They kept referring to it as my 'surgery' whenever they did bring it up. They just didn't know how to deal with it."

As we said earlier, individual reactions to your loss vary tremendously. Try to keep in mind that a person's reaction to you is based on his or her underlying personality and experiences. Also, that his reactions to you are a reflection of his own way of coping with things, as well as of his own life experiences. For example, one woman explains her sister-in-law's behavior the following way: "My sister-in-law was sympathetic and visited me when I was home, but the miscarriage occurred at an extremely stressful time for her — starting a new job — so she was preoccupied with that and had very little time for me."

Your loss may trigger feelings in friends and family members that cause them to be upset and confused. They may have a difficult time coping with their own painful feelings as well as with yours. In addition, they may be at a loss to know what to say to you. Rather than say the wrong thing, they may feel it best to say nothing at all. You may interpret their silence to mean they don't care when, in fact, they care so much they fear hurting you further.

On the other hand, you may find some people who don't understand what you are going through. If they have no interest in having children, they may not comprehend why you feel so badly. They have no sense of your yearning for a child, so they can't grasp your disappointment. Couples who have succeeded easily in having children and take pregnancy and birth for granted may not understand your frustration and pain, yet others with children may comprehend your grief completely. Although they had no problems, they fully appreciate the joys of parenthood. They are sensitive enough to feel hurt and disturbed that you have been denied what they find so fulfilling. They need only put themselves in your place and imagine the horror it would have been if they had lost their baby.

Another group of parents may react in a different way. They have children but are unhappy as parents. Some may be sorry they ever had children and feel that you are better off to have lost your baby. Their pregnancies might have been accidental, or regretted. These feelings are not easy to admit to oneself and even harder to confess to someone else, but they may be present in some of the people you know, and this may influence the way they deal with you.

Friends who are pregnant may worry that they, too, will lose their baby. Even a couple contemplating pregnancy may be fearful. When a friend or relative loses a baby, the saying "It can't happen to me" loses some of its credibility. Years after the birth of her son, one woman told her cousin: "Before you lost your baby, I never thought those things *really* happened. When I became pregnant, I worried constantly that my baby would die, as yours did. My fear was particularly strong in my eighth month, since your baby died then, so unexpectedly. I had a whole different way of thinking about my pregnancy because of what happened to you. I was terrified." A couple who is expecting a child may find it too anxiety-provoking to see you and may cope by avoiding you. This doesn't mean they are not sympathetic or don't care, but that they are scared it might happen to them and don't want to be reminded of the possibility.

Your pregnancy loss may evoke in others fear that might not be limited to issues regarding pregnancy. The death of your baby, although it was unborn, is a death nonetheless. Some people use denial and avoidance to cope with the issue of death. Hearing you discuss how badly you feel may be both painful and threatening for them. Your mourning may remind them that they and those around them are vulnerable to death at any time — they cannot control its inevitability. Rather than face these disconcerting feelings, they may stay away completely or avoid discussing your loss with you. It may be difficult for you to accept such avoidance behavior from family members and friends. There are times when our needs conflict with the needs of those we care about. Maybe there will be a change with time, and the relationship will survive, but it may not.

EXPECTANT GRANDPARENTS

Some reactions of family members may be based solely on the unique nature of family relationships. In many families, the parents of the couple who lost the baby were devastated by the news. They were sad watching their children suffering, knowing the tremendous impact of the loss on their lives. In addition, the loss of their grandchild-to-be was painful for them, because they, too, had been anticipating the new addition to the family. They, too, had fantasies and were terribly disappointed. To some, the child would have been their child as well — their second chance to be parents, particularly if they had no other grandchildren. In addition, the baby may have represented a new lease on life for them, or an exciting change, as they faced the onset of old age. Mothers often reexperience both their own pregnancies and their wish for a child when their daughters become pregnant. After the loss, they may feel personally deprived, aware of how the child would have touched their own life.

Because grandparents-to-be often experience a personal loss when their child's pregnancy fails, they may experience some of the same emotional reactions that their children are feeling —

pain, sadness, emptiness, anger and disappointment. These feelings are intensified by the fact that their children are hurting. They mourn with their children and they mourn for themselves.

HELP OTHERS TO HELP YOU

Other people sometimes don ι understand what they can do for you to help you feel better. Don't assume they understand the depths of your loss, particularly if they haven't been through the experience themselves.

It is best to assume that your friends and family may want to do the right thing but do not know what the right thing is. Not everyone instinctively knows what you want. The first thing to do is figure out for yourself what you want from people, then tell them your wishes.

You may have friends or family members who are afraid to ask about your feelings, wishing to avoid opening a Pandora's box for your sake, when you would like nothing more than to pour your heart out. You may need to initiate the discussion. Give them a chance to be there for you, if this is so. This is a time to strengthen bonds with friends and relatives.

If you are especially sensitive to the things people say to you, tell them if they are hurting your feelings. If hearing "It happened for the best" upsets you, let people know. They probably have put themselves in your place and are saying what they would like to hear. A simple explanation of your feelings should set things straight: "I understand you're trying to be helpful, but I can't accept the idea that it happened for the best at this time. It only makes me feel worse. I'm grieving for my lost baby."

There may be some practical things you would like your friends and family to do for you. It is likely they will be more than happy to help. Possibly you need help with shopping, cooking, or cleaning, or you may feel that you need to rest, or that you need time alone. If you have other children, you may need someone to help you with child care from time to time. Whenever possible tell people who wish to help you how they can be most helpful to you. They will feel better if they can do something for you, and chances are you will feel better, too.

IV.

Planning for the Future

Under the best of circumstances, it is extremely difficult to deal with the loss of a desired pregnancy. Hopes are shattered and faith in your own body may be badly damaged. In addition, you must face the frustration of not being able to control your destiny, whether on the level of being able to set a schedule for achieving certain life goals, or even for being able to have the things you want.

The loss of your pregnancy has probably caused a major disruption in your plans. From the moment you found out you were pregnant, all of your plans centered around the pregnancy and the expectation that you would have a baby.

You may have planned your career around the upcoming birth, stopped working or cut back in order to get ready for the baby. You may have made arrangements for a leave of absence from your job, or decided to stay at home indefinitely with your baby. If you have not been working, you may have modified your usual activities in anticipation of having a baby.

When you were pregnant, you may have bought or made maternity or baby clothes and picked out birth announcements. Friends and family may have worked away feverishly to have everything ready for your due date. You may have envisioned how "big" you would be by Thanksgiving, that you would feel the baby kick by your husband's birthday, and that you would be "waddling around" by the first of April.

Then, in one moment, all your dreams and plans were shot to hell. There was no baby, not this time.

You are faced with an awesome and overwhelming task. You must deal with your grief and at the same time reorient yourself to the reality of not being pregnant and not having the baby you yearn for.

It is not going to be easy to cope with the emptiness and pain; they will be with you for a long time. Try to accept that they cannot be erased.

How do you put together the pieces of your life when you are paralyzed with grief and unable to know what the future holds in store? There are no simple answers to this question. Each couple must travel the lonely road back from despair in their own time and in their own way. Each must confront many painful feelings, overcome them, and eventually lay them to rest. Then, and only then, will they be ready to go on with their lives.

The loss of your pregnancy has no doubt affected you emotionally, and perhaps physically as well. Because this has happened to you, decisions that you made in the past may no longer be desirable or feasible. Among the most important choices that will be facing you is whether you still want a child or whether you want to remain childless. If you decide that you want a child, you must then ask yourself whether you wish to become pregnant again, if you wish to adopt, or if you would like to pursue both possibilities simultaneously. The decision that you reach should be based on many considerations: what the chances are that you will be able to become pregnant, or that a new pregnancy will be successful; if you are feeling ready to cope with the stress of being pregnant again; what medical risks you face if you decide to become pregnant; how much you want to have a child; how long you are willing to wait to have a child; if adoption is a possible alternative for you; and how flexible you are about the type of child you would be willing to take.

After thinking about these issues, and discussing them between yourselves and with your physician, you must make a decision. You may decide to try again, even if the odds for success are not great, or the risk to your health is significant. Although there may be some possibility that you could have a successful pregnancy if you tried again, you may not be willing to take the emotional or physical risks involved. You may decide that you prefer to remain childless or you may elect to adopt. Possibly you do not feel ready to make any decision for a while. You may be feeling depleted and in need of time to recover before tackling something new, or you may be feeling too vulnerable to plunge into a pregnancy right now. The choice about how to proceed is a personal one.

8. Choosing to Try Again

Most of you will make the decision to try to become pregnant again. This is a successful coping mechanism because it has the potential to give you what you want most: a baby. Once you have made this decision you will need to think about how long you want to wait before trying to become pregnant. We suggest that you examine the following considerations.

MEDICAL CONSIDERATIONS

There is some controversy among physicians about what is the optimal time to wait before trying to conceive again. It is generally felt that the likelihood of miscarriage is diminished if conception is not attempted until the woman has had three normal menstrual periods. However, a minority of physicians feel that such a long time is not necessary, and that if the woman is anxious to become pregnant again, she may attempt conception after having one normal menstrual period. Since controversy exists about this matter, you will want to base your decision on your physician's recommendation, as well as on your own inclination.

Regardless of what time period is actually decided upon, you may be faced with the urge not to wait. A strong desire to become pregnant immediately may overshadow your rational decision. You may throw caution to the wind and attempt to become pregnant as soon as possible. Alternatively, you may choose to resist temptation because you want to do everything in your power to make your next pregnancy successful. Some couples chose to wait before trying again, because they believe that if they don't, and then lose their next pregnancy, they will blame themselves. This, too, should be taken into consideration in making your decision.

PSYCHOLOGICAL CONSIDERATIONS

There is some controversy about the length of time one should let pass before one is psychologically ready to try again. There are those who believe that a couple should wait six months to a year before conceiving or adopting. This recommendation is based on concern that unless they have sufficient time to mourn the child they lost, a second child may be regarded as a replacement. It is generally believed that in order for each child to be dealt with as a separate and unique individual, the parents' mourning process must be completed. Otherwise there is risk of contaminating the relationship with future children with unresolved feelings and fantasies about the child who was lost. It is also important for the couple to consider whether or not they feel ready to face trying again, and whether they feel ready to deal with the stress of another pregnancy.

We have found that the optimal time to wait before trying again is an individual matter and depends on one's own personality structure, past experiences, motivation to be a parent, and support network. It has been our experience that what is critical is that one has mourned one's loss, not how long a time period actually passes before a new pregnancy is attempted.

THE WAITING PERIOD

Most physicians recommend the use of a mechanical method of birth control (such as condoms, a diaphragm, or foam) during the waiting period. Like many couples, you may find it painful and ironic to have to use birth control at a time when you strongly desire to be pregnant. You may also find that mechanical methods of birth control are inconvenient and that they interrupt spontaneous lovemaking. Each time you make love you are faced with the decision of using or not using contraception. This conflict may trigger painful feelings all over again.

During the waiting period you will probably anticipate what it will be like when you begin trying to get pregnant. You may feel hopeful and optimistic, eagerly await each menstrual period, and count the days until you can try again. Or possibly you may feel anxious to try again, but extremely fearful that you will not be able to conceive. If you have a history of infertility, this fear may be intensified.

TRYING AGAIN

When the waiting is over and the time to try again finally arrives, you may find yourself in an emotional state you did not anticipate. You may have conflicting feelings: the fear of *not becoming* pregnant and the fear of *becoming* pregnant. In addition, the fears you had when you were waiting to try may be accentuated now that the possibility of pregnancy is closer at hand. You may be preoccupied with becoming pregnant to the exclusion of everything in your life. You may find yourself living by the menstrual cycle and you may find that your entire existence is focused on becoming pregnant. If you have had an infertility problem, you may discover that many of your feelings are familiar.

During the fertile time of the month you may find yourself obsessed with becoming pregnant. You may fantasize where the egg is each hour, not wanting to lose your chance. Now is the time to have intercourse whether or not you feel like it. You are motivated to have sex, not for pleasure but for procreation. This may lead to sexual difficulties such as refusal to "perform," performance anxiety, or decreased libido. As you approach the end of your cycle you may feel both anxious and hopeful that you won't have to go through another month of this. You may be preoccupied with searching for signs and symptoms of early pregnancy.

Marion was thirty-eight years old when she became pregnant for the first time. She had been trying for two years. She miscarried at nine weeks and decided to attempt another pregnancy four months later, partially because of her age. She told us that she was obsessed with becoming pregnant and that all else in her life had lost its meaning. She speaks of her behavior during this time: "Each month I spent one week constantly touching my breasts to see if they were sore like the first time I was pregnant and hoping they would hurt. For several days before my period was due, I ran to the bathroom every hour, praying there would be no blood."

If your period arrives, you feel angry, frustrated, and in despair. The first day of your menstrual period is most likely to be the worst of the month. Another month has gone by without success, and you start to wonder if you'll ever get pregnant again.

The cycle repeats itself as you gear up for the next try. As ovulation approaches, you put aside your disappointment and get ready to try again.

BEING PREGNANT AGAIN

"Congratulations! You are pregnant." Those magic words! This is the moment you have been waiting for, and you feel ecstatic. After what have seemed to you like endless months of waiting, your prayers have been answered. You want to shout out your news; you feel like phoning up everyone you know to tell them. But you don't — something holds you back.

Better be cautious; better not tell anyone until you are sure, you tell yourself. Within minutes you discover that this pregnancy is simply not going to be like your first.

What makes this time different is that you have lost your innocence. This time you are aware of all the things that can go wrong. You know that if it happened once, it could happen again. Although you want to relax and enjoy being pregnant, anxiety keeps getting in your way. Sometimes the pregnancy feels like a nightmare, full of fear and remembrances of your previous pregnancy. Many women find that they are eternally vigilant — every twinge, pain, or cramp is noted, amplified, and feared.

We talked to Julie before the birth of her son. She was eight months pregnant. Even though her chances of carrying this baby to term were excellent, she was still suffering from the trauma of her first experience. She had lost her first baby a year earlier in her sixth month. No reason for the stillbirth was diagnosed. Julie described her constant state of fear: "The first six months of *this* pregnancy I was terrified. I kept dreaming of my labor and delivery, the doctor was saying, 'You're gonna lose it.' " I dreaded going to the bathroom for fear there would be blood. I always felt reassured when my breasts were sore. I wanted this baby more than anything in the world, and because I wanted it so much, I felt sure that something would go wrong. At the beginning I spent endless hours imagining things that could go wrong — I would convince myself that I didn't have a chance. Every time I felt a twinge of pain I would feel hysterical inside. I lost my ability to tell which pains were normal and which weren't — everything felt the same to me — anything could mean the end of all of my hopes.

"I must have called my doctor a dozen times to tell him about one concern or another. Usually he would tell me not to worry. However, if I was really frantic he would always see me. Luckily, he never found anything to worry about, and I was always able to leave his office somewhat reassured. Unfortunately, my feelings of wellbeing never lasted very long. Within a few days, I would find something else to worry about.

"I think I almost drove my husband crazy. Sometimes it got so bad that I would convince him that there really was something wrong with the baby. Those times were the worst. Even though I am in my eighth month, I'm still terrified. I can't forget what I went through and I live in constant fear of it happening again this time. I probably won't rest until the baby is in my arms."

Even when things do go well, it may be hard to enjoy being pregnant. This can be a frustrating experience. You wish you could be as blissfully oblivious as other pregnant women. You yearn to be able to enjoy being pregnant, the way other women do — it doesn't seem fair to have this spoiled also. Unfortunately, if you have ever had the experience of losing a pregnancy, pregnancy probably will never again be a state of bliss for you. With luck, there will be many happy moments. It is likely that there will also be some tense or anxious ones, not because anything will necessarily go wrong, but because it is hard not to imagine the worst sometimes. Some women have likened the experience of losing a pregnancy to the way they felt the first time someone they knew had died. Before someone you actually know dies, you know about death, but it doesn't really have an impact on you. Death is something that happens to people out there, not to anyone in your world. Beforehand, death is an abstract concept, without any real meaning. Afterward, life feels incredibly fragile, and you realize how very vulnerable you are. The same seems to hold true for pregnancy.

Before you actually lost a pregnancy, you probably knew that some pregnancies were unsuccessful. However, if you were like most women, you probably didn't give this much thought. Since it happened to you, your fear of losing a pregnancy is probably much greater. Rationally you know that most pregnancies are successful; still, it is difficult not to feel anxious. Once you lose your innocence, there is no way of getting it back. You have been changed by your experience, and will never be the same again.

A Precious Pregnancy

If you have lost a pregnancy, it is doubtful that you will ever take being pregnant for granted. This has both its good side and its more problematic side. On the positive side, it is likely that you will truly value being pregnant and will have an appreciation of the miracle that is unfolding inside you. This would not have been as possible had you not experienced the pain you have been through. For you, pregnancy will never be just something that is going on in your body while the rest of you is occupied with more important things. Similarly, there is little danger that you will miss one precious moment, that even the smallest new development will pass unnoticed, or that you will fail to set aside time to appreciate the experience fully.

On the problematic side is the anxiety that almost always accompanies a particularly "precious" pregnancy. This is no ordinary pregnancy for you. This is the pregnancy that you have been hoping for and dreaming of. If you are like most women who have once lost a pregnancy, you are not about to do the slightest thing to endanger it. Not for you the advice that "pregnancy is a natural state; you need not curtail your usual activities, unless they are particularly strenuous or dangerous." The moment you find out that you are pregnant, you feel like a fragile vessel carrying an even more fragile cargo. Rationally you know that a normal pregnancy is quite impervious to bumps, jumps, and even falls. However, you may decide that although this might be true for other women, you prefer to play it safe. If you have questions about what activities are permissible, ask your physician for his opinion. If he does not

feel that you need to restrict your activities, your personal preference can be your guide. You should do only what you feel psychologically and physically comfortable doing.

Expecting Too Much

"This is the pregnancy you have been looking forward to, and now
that it is a reality, you'd better enjoy every moment of it." "This is
a precious moment in your life, and you'd better cherish it."
Thoughts like these are commonly experienced by pregnant
women who have lived through infertility, losing a pregnancy, or
both. Noble sentiments; however, not totally realistic. Pregnancy,
under the best of circumstances, can have its less appealing side.
Fatigue, nausea, and vomiting are common in the first trimester,
while a variety of aches and pains, exhaustion, urinary frequency,
and trouble getting around often bother even the heartiest of souls
during the third trimester. Not you, however; you are supposed to
be grateful that you are pregnant, and you don't have the right to
complain about any part of it. If a complaint manages to sneak
out, you feel guilty — after all this was what you wanted, wasn't
it? After wanting to be pregnant so badly, you probably feel that it
is unreasonable of you to have negative feelings about any part
of it.

Often when we very much want something that is not immediately available to us, we create fantasies of what it would be like to
have our wish come true. These fantasies are usually a highly ideal-
ized, and therefore unrealistic, version of the real thing. The problem is that often the real thing is not quite as good as the fantasy:
that is, it is not as good as you imagined it would be. When we
imagine what being pregnant will be like, we think of a rounded
belly, full breasts, ourselves proudly wearing maternity clothes,
and a beaming husband. Endless mornings of nausea, sleepiness,
and anxiety just aren't what dreams are made of, yet for many
women, this is what pregnancy is apt to be like.

A word of caution: in the same way that your fantasies of what
pregnancy would be like may have led you to have unrealistic expectations about the experience, and of yourself as a pregnant
woman, your fantasies about what it will be like to have a baby
and to be a mother may leave you ill prepared for dealing with the

less glorious aspects of that experience. Both pregnancy and motherhood can be pleasurable and fulfilling; they can also be difficult and frustrating, especially when you feel that there is something wrong with you for feeling that you should not have any negative feelings.

Holding Back

Fear of losing another baby inhibits many couples from emotionally investing in the next pregnancy. They know that loss can happen again, and so try to protect themselves in case it does. Often, they allow themselves little, if any, bonding with the baby during pregnancy. Some say that "holding back" was their way of protecting themselves from feeling completely devastated should this pregnancy also fail.

Even when things go well, and the pregnancy progresses normally, it may be difficult to invest your love and hope. Julie, whom we spoke about a while earlier, found it difficult to allow herself to feel attached to her unborn child, not because she didn't love it, but because she wanted it so badly. "I never really let myself enjoy being pregnant. I held my feelings back the entire time. I tried not to let myself think about a baby — in fact, I almost managed to disconnect being pregnant from having a baby. It was almost as if, if I relaxed and allowed myself to believe that I really was going to have a child, something would come along and take it all away. I know that I was protecting myself from feeling too disappointed had anything gone wrong. Last time I was so devastated that, no matter what, I didn't want to ever feel that way again. I guess that my husband felt the same way, because we seemed to have an unspoken agreement that this time we would not let our hopes grow. I think that in some ways we both were emotionally frozen throughout the pregnancy."

Julie and her husband decided not to let their friends and family know about the pregnancy until her sixth month was completed. They felt that they would be tempting fate to announce it before then. They also felt that they would be less disappointed if the pregnancy was lost before everyone knew about it. Julie's reluctance to let people know is not unusual; many couples who have lost pregnancies choose to do the same. Some say that they felt too vulnerable to let other people know, others felt that by not telling they could protect families and friends from feeling disappointed. Even couples who do not hold off telling others as long as Julie did, often wait until the end of the third month to let people know, since the major danger of losing the pregnancy is over by then.

Although there is usually no rational cause for concern, many women find that they are unable to enjoy their pregnancies until they have passed the month when their first babies died. Often after this point their anxiety subsides. Many hold off telling people that they are pregnant and wearing maternity clothes until the "magic" month has passed. Charlotte, the relieved mother of a beautiful three-month-old girl, reflected back on her most recent pregnancy. Her first baby died at the seventh month for unknown reasons.

"I was very scared during my first seven months that I would lose my baby again. I took extra good care of myself: resting, eating well. After I passed my seventh month I decided to be happy and enjoy being pregnant. I had gotten robbed the first time and was determined to make it up. I made my mind up that I would deal with the loss if and when it happened.

"Early on, my husband and doctor were the only people who knew I was pregnant again. I did not tell anyone until I was obviously showing or they asked outright. I was too afraid this one would die too and I'd have to explain it all over again. I held off buying maternity clothes as long as I could, then I bought them piece by piece. I didn't want to buy a lot of things and then have no reason to wear them. I had thrown away all my old maternity clothes after I lost my last baby because I couldn't bear to look at them. I felt it would be bad luck to wear them this time.

"Only after my seventh month passed did I feel safe enough to buy any baby clothes or start furnishing the nursery. I even started to believe that I was really going to have a baby."

Waiting for the Results of Amniocentesis
Couples who anticipate having to have an amniocentesis often find themselves unable to feel a sense of relief until they have obtained the test results and learned that all is well. Amniocentesis is a procedure that has been available in recent years for determining

whether the fetus has any one of a number of genetic or metabolic conditions. It is usually recommended for all women who are thirty-five or older. This is because women over the age of thirty-five have a significantly increased risk of producing a child with Down's syndrome (also known as mongolism or trisomy 21). Women under thirty have approximately one chance in 1,500 of having a child with Down's syndrome. The incidence of this disease increases markedly with the mother's age, so that the chance that a woman between the ages of thirty and thirty-four will have an afflicted child is 1 in 750. Between thirty-five and thirty-nine the incidence is about 1 in 300, and between forty and forty-four it is approximately 1 in 80.

Amniocentesis is also recommended to parents of any age if they have produced a child with a genetic defect, if they have produced a child who has an inherited metabolic disorder, such as Tay-Sachs disease or Gaucher's disease, or if they themselves are either carriers of these conditions, have a family history of inherited disease, or are themselves affected. For example, a couple whose family is known to carry a sex-linked chromosomal disorder such as hemophilia or Duchenne muscular dystrophy should have an amniocentesis performed.

The actual procedure in an amniocentesis is very simple. Sometime between the fifteenth and seventeenth week of gestation, a procedure known as ultrasound scanning, which uses high-frequency sound waves to visualize the fetus, the placenta, and the amniotic cavity, is used to pinpoint these structures. Using local anesthesia, a needle is inserted through the pregnant woman's abdomen into the amniotic sac, and a small amount of yellowish amniotic fluid is drawn off. This fluid contains some fetal cells. Samples of the amniotic fluid are then sent to the laboratory for study. The fetal cells are incubated, and when they have reproduced sufficiently, they are subjected to a number of tests. It usually takes several weeks until there are a sufficient number of cells so that tests can be done. The amniotic fluid itself is analyzed for the presence of a specific protein, alpha-fetoprotein, unusually high concentrations of which can indicate that the fetus has an open neural tube defect.

If indicated, other specific tests can be done to determine

whether the fetus has any one of several biochemical abnormalities, which could cause a metabolic disease (for instance, lack of the enzyme hexosaminidase A indicates presence of Tay-Sachs disease), or whether an inherited sex-linked disease such as hemophilia can be diagnosed.

Lastly, cells are isolated from the tissue culture, specially stained, and then viewed under electron microscope, to determine whether the fetus has any chromosomal abnormalities, such as Down's syndrome.

The weeks between the time when the amniocentesis is done and the final tests are completed are difficult ones for most couples, The test results will indicate if, as far as could be ascertained, the fetus is normal or whether a defective fetus has been discovered. In the latter situation, which occurs in a minority of cases, it is still early enough in the pregnancy for a safe therapeutic abortion to be performed.

Because the continuation of the pregnancy is contingent on the outcome of the amniocentesis, many couples find it difficult to invest themselves in the pregnancy until they are certain that it will not have to be interrupted. One veteran of two amniocenteses described feeling as if her emotions were suspended until she learned that each fetus was normal. Only after obtaining the report indicating that all was well was she able to let herself form an attachment to her future child. This woman's experience is fairly typical. No matter how optimistic one is, it is the rare couple that does not breathe a sigh of relief when the test results come back indicating that no abnormalities were found.

WHEN YOUR BABY ARRIVES

Parents who have lost a pregnancy often find that although the birth of a child eases their pain greatly, it does not erase it entirely. They discover that there is no starting afresh, that the memory of what they have been through stays with them and affects them in many ways.

Commonly, couples who have experienced the loss of a pregnancy protect themselves from becoming too attached to subsequent pregnancies. One effect of this may be that for them the bonding process to their child begins at birth, rather than beforehand. Also, since they may not have allowed themselves to think very much about what it would be like to be a parent or to take care of a child, they may find themselves less psychologically prepared for their new role than are couples who have spent the pregnancy anticipating what would be expected of them. As a consequence, they may find that for a brief time after their baby's birth they can't quite believe that they actually have a child and that they are its parents. These feelings are experienced by many new parents and are nothing to be concerned about. Fortunately love develops quickly, as do caretaking skills, and within a few days or weeks it feels as if the baby has always been theirs.

It is also likely that the baby born of a "precious pregnancy" will be a very precious baby. It is to be hoped that this will only heighten your delight in your new child: this is your "miracle" child, the child you feared might never happen, and everything about him or her will probably feel quite special. It is also possible that the "specialness" of this child for you may make you feel overly concerned about his or her wellbeing or about your parenting ability.

People who have always had a predisposition to worry tend to be particularly vulnerable to this type of anxiety. A recent encounter with the cruelty of fate seems to reinforce their feelings of vulnerability: they fear that if something bad has happened to them once, it could happen again. While this fear is understandable, it is important to remember that just because you feel particularly vulnerable doesn't mean that you actually are. Most couples find that as time passes their anxiety gradually lessens. If you find that this is not so for you, counseling may be useful in helping you put the past in perspective, so that you can more fully enjoy being a parent.

It is also important to keep in mind that even the most special and long-awaited baby may at times be less than a total delight. There is a tendency among parents who have lost a pregnancy to feel that they are being ungrateful if they are ever tired, overworked, or short-tempered. After all, this is the baby they have been looking forward to for so long — what's wrong with them, they ask themselves, for sometimes feeling exhausted or upset? While it is normal to feel that not all aspects of being a parent are pleasurable, parents who have experienced pregnancy loss tend not to give themselves permission to have anything other than positive feelings. As a result, they often feel guilty and inadequate, although there is no real reason for feeling that way. This attitude may be compounded when friends and family members are insensitive to what the new parents are experiencing, and when they add their overblown expectations to the couple's own.

There is a tendency in our society to believe that a lost pregnancy can be replaced by a new one and that the scars that one develops when one loses a pregnancy are eradicated by the birth of a new baby. Most couples find that their experience is not quite so simple. Some couples may find that the birth of a child reopens old wounds, because it so vividly reminds them of what they had lost. While the birth of a child goes a long way toward alleviating the pain they feel, it does not do away with it entirely. There will always be feelings of regret at what could have been, as well as painful memories of what they had been through.

9. Choosing Childlessness

Once upon a time you made the decision to have children. When you made this decision, chances are that you assumed that if you wanted to have children you would be able to without difficulty. When things did not work out as you planned, you were forced to reconsider the options available to you.

The decision to remain childless comes about in different ways for different couples. Some couples discover that while they were willing to go ahead with having a child if it could be done easily, they were not willing to make the effort to have one if it meant enduring an infertility evaluation and medical treatment; the physical, emotional, and financial costs of continuing to try; the frustration and pain of enduring multiple losses; or the effort to pursue adoption.

Some couples have found that the experience of being pregnant and losing a pregnancy has helped them recognize that childbearing was not for them. One or both partners may have found that they experienced doubts or negative feelings during the pregnancy. We picture pregnancy as a time of excitement and happiness, but it can also be a time of stress and uncertainty if one partner or both have doubts about whether they want to have children. The woman may find that being pregnant brings into focus many apprehensions. She may fear that if she has a child she will lose her freedom, or she may feel that having a child will bring about a drastic change in her responsibilities, whether she becomes a homemaker or continues working. She may feel she has to give up quite a lot in order to rear a child and may be unsure if she wants to make that commitment. The man may also be sensitive to the responsibility a child will bring, as well as to the change in lifestyle that having a child will bring about. He may be concerned that he will come second to a child in his wife's affections, or he may worry about the financial obligations involved in raising a child.

Sometimes couples choose to remain childless because they are unable to produce their own biological child, although they would have liked to; and one or both partners do not wish to adopt. When partners are in agreement about what they want, things usually work out well. More problematic are situations where one spouse wishes to adopt and the other does not wish to. This latter situation may leave one or both partners feeling angry, frustrated, or depressed, and when unresolved may cause major marital problems or even the breakup of the marriage.

Other couples remain childless, although they would like to have a child and would happily adopt one, either because they were not accepted by an agency, because they were not eligible to adopt the kind of child they were hoping for, because they were unable to find a child that they could adopt privately, or because private adoption is illegal in their state.

Childless living can be a positive choice; as such it can be both satisfying and rewarding. Increasing numbers of couples are choosing not to have children. Couples who have made this choice feel that it affords them many advantages.

The couple who does not have children can choose to live life free of many of the constraints that influence couples with children. They can live and work in ways that suit themselves, but that might not be compatible with the needs of a child. Choices vary from options such as working long hours, pursuing a demanding career, or returning to school to earn a degree, all of which can be done with less trouble without a child than with one, to such unconventional options as pursuing work that one loves but that does not pay well, or traveling to remote areas of the globe for long or short periods of time. In almost every realm of their lives the couple without children has more freedom than do couples with children. For the most part they need pay attention to their own needs alone. This can mean going out to a movie or away for the weekend without making complicated arrangements, sleeping late without interruption, or having free time available for sports, visiting with friends, being together, or just doing nothing.

In addition, the couple who does not have children need provide financially only for themselves, and so may enjoy a larger share of whatever economic resources are available to them than would be the case if they had a child to feed, clothe, and shelter, not to mention to send to college. Inflation has made it difficult for the average family to get by with one salary; as a consequence many couples are choosing to have both partners work outside the home. In many areas child-care services do not meet the need for them, and when available are often quite costly. Without this support a couple's ability to both work and raise children may be severely compromised, perhaps making it necessary to choose between the two. When one adds the cost of raising a child to the age of eighteen in the United States, estimated by the Population Reference Bureau as somewhere between $40,000 and $65,000 dollars, not counting the cost of college, it is not difficult to see why, for many couples, having children is a major economic burden.

In recent years, as women have entered the labor force in increasing numbers, many have found that their primary satisfaction could be derived from work, and that they neither needed nor wanted the added responsibility of having a child. Similarly, as women have been accepted into professional schools and career training programs in ever-increasing numbers and the possibilities for having a successful career have expanded, more women are electing to pursue career choices that either preclude entirely or make very difficult having a child.

Choosing not to have children of one's own need not mean that one must live a life without children. There are many ways for those who desire contact with children to bring this about. Teaching has long been a way for people who enjoy being with children to play a meaningful part in their lives. Working in a school as a nurse, maintenance person, dietitian, or secretary can yield similar benefits. So too can volunteer work with hospitalized, institutionalized, bedridden, or handicapped children, whose lives could be greatly improved by a relationship with a caring adult. Leading a Girl Scout or Boy Scout troop, being a Big Brother or Big Sister to a child, befriending neighborhood children, volunteering at a day-care center or becoming a special aunt or uncle to a niece or nephew are other possible ways to enrich your own life, as well as the lives of those who are lucky enough to have you for a friend.

One can choose to have as much or as little contact with children as one desires. Being foster parents to several children can totally fill your life; working for a cause that will ultimately benefit children can be far less time-consuming, but enormously gratifying, nonetheless. In short, the possibilities for having children in your life are many. The world is full of children to share and to love even if you don't bear or adopt your own.

As social pressure to conform to one acceptable lifestyle decreases, more and more people are exploring new alternatives. Child-free marriage is slowly and steadily gaining public acceptance as traditional ideas about what constitutes a family are expanded. The couple who chooses not to have children need no longer hide in the closet. Increasingly, groups such as ZPG (Zero Population Growth) and National Alliance for Optional Parenthood are serving as both a support group and as an advocate for couples who choose to remain childless.

The following is a description of one couple's route to choosing childlessness.

"After four years of trying to conceive and then two miscarriages, my husband and I decided to quit trying, but we hadn't given up on the idea of raising children. We had been through infertility testing and had conceived both times through artificial insemination (with my husband Steve's sperm). The problem was that my cervical mucus was hostile to Steve's sperm. We were very excited with the first pregnancy and crushed when it ended at about three months. We became less excited over the second pregnancy — I miscarried a week after the pregnancy test, at two and a half months.

"After the second loss, I kept telling myself we could try again, that there was hope, but I was also afraid of more disappointment. My age, thirty-eight, was uppermost in my mind — we couldn't keep trying for years on end. And the years of ups and downs of trying and hoping were taking a toll. I was edgy, easily depressed, and Steve, who had always been very patient and calm, was irritable. About a month after the second miscarriage, we had a long talk about our feelings and coping or lack of coping with our situation. "Do we really want to stay on this roller coaster?" Steve asked. I started to cry at the thought of giving up, but I had to admit that I longed to return to our normal life. My life had become centered on getting pregnant. I worked as a legal secretary, but felt I was only marking time until I could become a full-time mother. It was hard to face the fact that we might not have a child, as we had dreamed for so long. Steve and I agreed that night that we would think about other possibilities — adoption and childlessness. We had both been married previously and neither Steve nor I had children from those marriages. We realized we were getting old to have children and after seven years of marriage, a baby would be a big adjustment.

"I wasn't ready to give up entirely, though, and started looking into adoption. We went to an information meeting on adoption held by our county's social service department and found that only older children, not infants, were available. We felt inadequate to cope with a six-year-old who had lived in various foster homes. We felt discouraged. Then I contacted adoption agencies and heard there was a three- to five-year wait. Adoption didn't seem a good alternative for us — at our age we felt we couldn't wait and we doubted whether agencies would even accept our application. Wouldn't they be more likely to place babies with thirty-year-olds?

"We pondered adoption for a number of weeks and gradually decided against pursuing it. Then we just drifted for a while, several months at least, only occasionally discussing our quandary. I still wanted to be around kids, and a few months later an opportunity arose. Our church needed an elementary Sunday School teacher, so I volunteered. That was over a year ago. Steve helps with the class of about twenty youngsters, and we enjoy it very much.

"Over the last year since we decided to think about other possibilities than having our own children, we have become more relaxed. Our acceptance of our loss of our dream to have children was gradual. The reality of the situation slowly seeped in.

"My work means much more to me now and I'm taking classes

to become a paralegal assistant. I'm developing a positive attitude about not having children, though there still is a pang at times.

"We have a good life together and are happier now that the stress of trying to conceive is gone. Nearly every Saturday or Sunday we go hiking, sometimes alone and sometimes with a club we belong to. We've found that our life is full."

10. Deciding to Adopt

If you are not able to conceive, if you are unable to carry a pregnancy successfully to term, or if you are unwilling to attempt another pregnancy because of either the physical or the emotional risk involved, and if you strongly desire to have a child and to experience parenthood, adoption is worth considering.

Perhaps the most significant aspect of the decision to adopt is that it is a "decision." Adoption is not the automatic, obvious way for most couples to fill the empty cradle in the nursery. Couples do not adopt by merely leading their normal lives and leaving things up to nature. In order for an adoption to happen, one must make a concerted effort to bring it about.

The process by which one decides whether or not to pursue adoption and the factors influencing the timing of this process are different for each couple. In part, how one proceeds is determined by where one begins. The couple who is certain that they will never be able to bear their own child may see adoption as offering them their only chance for having a child in their lives, whereas the couple who still has the potential ability to produce their own biological child, despite several unsuccessful pregnancies, may see adoption as an option for the future, rather than something they wish to consider for the present. The couple who has always considered adopting a child will find the idea less foreign than will the couple who has never considered the possibility. Most couples consider adopting a child when their own attempts at having a child have been unsuccessful. However, not everyone draws the line in the same place. Some couples are able to keep trying and to feel optimistic about their chances of success, despite many losses, while others decide to give up trying to have their own child after one or two unsuccessful pregnancies.

Each couple has to figure out when to begin the adoption process. This decision is easier for those who know that they are unable to have children. They are more likely to begin immediately after deciding that they wish to adopt.

On the other hand, couples who have experienced one or more unsuccessful pregnancies may still have the ability, albeit theoretical, to produce a child themselves. This group faces the most complex decision, since, as is so often true in life, they must base their deliberations on supposition rather than on fact. If four pregnancies have been unsuccessful, who is to say that the same will or will not hold true for the fifth pregnancy? When does it make sense to stop trying? Would one more try result in the birth of a much-desired child? If you have had one ectopic pregnancy, will the second pregnancy be different? Unfortunately, there is no way of predicting what the answers to these questions will be.

Since it is not possible to read the future, whatever decision is made must be based on either intuition, an overriding preference, or on a careful assessment of one's situation. If you have an intuitive sense of how to proceed, or if you *know* how you want to go about becoming parents, your path is before you. If, however, you are uncertain about whether or not you are ready to adopt, it may be helpful to weigh the following factors. First, with the help of your physician you should try to assess the likelihood that you will be able to carry a pregnancy successfully to term, and produce a healthy child. As one would guess, the prognosis for a successful pregnancy is different for the couple who has had a long history of fetal deaths and for the couple who has produced two children before having a single miscarriage. Your prognosis is dependent not only on your reproductive history; whether or not the cause of pregnancy loss has been determined may be of importance. If a treatable cause has been found, the odds of success may be different than if no cause has been found. Similarly, your current state of health needs to be taken into account in determining the prognosis for future pregnancies. Since some chronic diseases predispose to fetal loss, the woman who has such a condition needs to know if her current condition will negatively influence the outcome of a pregnancy.

Your age and that of your spouse are another factor that needs to enter into your decision-making process. If you are young, you have many years before you in which to keep trying, before your biological time clock is going to run out. On the other hand, if you are in your late thirties and have been trying for years to have a child without success, it is doubtful, but not impossible, that several more years of trying will bring success.

In addition, if you would like to be able to apply to an adoption agency, your age at the time you apply may determine both whether or not the agency considers you eligible and what type of placement they would consider you eligible for. Since the upper age limit that most agencies consider suitable for an infant placement is somewhere around forty years, you increase your chance of being successful if you apply before you reach this age.

Other factors to weigh in deciding whether or not to adopt or to attempt another pregnancy are whether a pregnancy would subject you to significant physical risk and/or whether a pregnancy is likely to result in the birth of a congenitally defective child. A woman who has narrowly escaped death when her tube burst may not be anxious to tempt fate. Similarly, women with medical conditions that increase in severity during pregnancy may well be inclined to avoid further problems. So, too, the couple who has given birth to a child with a congenital defect, especially if the presence of the defect cannot be determined by amniocentesis.

Some couples give up on trying to have a biological child and decide to adopt for other reasons. The wear and tear of years of trying may be significant, as may the feelings of disappointment and discouragement that result from it. It is not uncommon to feel that you just couldn't stand losing another pregnancy — that one more loss would do you in. Related to this is the desire for certainty that most couples have. Living with uncertainty can take its toll. In addition, coping with an uncertain future, especially when your desire for a child is strong, can be extremely stressful. Deciding to adopt is one way of eliminating the uncertainty that results from depending on one's own erratic biology.

The most important factor that leads many to adopt is the urgent desire to have a child. As one couple expressed this motivation: "We have lost valuable years, years when we would have liked to have had a child in our lives. I guess we could keep on trying to have our own, but who knows if we ever will, and even if we did eventually, who is to predict how many years from now that will be. I guess, neither of us are willing to take the chance that someday we might be successful."

One of the first things that most couples who have considered adoption realize is that adopting a child is not the same as producing one's own biological child. In order to determine whether adoption is right for you, you should ask yourself how you feel about some of the differences. Among the gratifications an adopted child cannot offer are the experience and satisfaction of creating a human being, the ability to enhance your marriage by producing a child with your spouse, the fulfillment of experiencing pregnancy and childbearing, and the security of being equal to and like your friends and relatives who have had their own biological children.

You must be able to come to terms with the loss of these "biological benefits" before you can completely accept adoption as an alternative. It is not easy for those of us who have spent our entire lives expecting that someday we would have a child of our own, to give up that goal.

Nevertheless, couples who recognize that their goal is to have a child in their lives, and who feel that this desire overshadows their need for a biological connection, are able to find fulfillment by adopting a child.

The realization that parenthood is one's primary goal does not, however, end the decision-making process. Other valid and important questions must be answered before an intelligent choice can be made. For example, the question "Can I love an adopted child?" must be confronted. One must examine one's need to love another, and understand it thoroughly, before one can comfortably and unambivalently say "Yes." It is also necessary to ask yourself what type of child you prefer, and how flexible you are able to be about what you could accept. Could you love an older child, a handicapped child, or a child of a different race, or is the only type of child you would consider adopting one that is similar to what you would have produced?

Another area that is worth some thought is how you feel about the "adoptive relationship." Are you worried that your child will not love you, because you did not give birth to him or her? Are you concerned about how to tell your child about his or her origins? Are you fearful that the child's biological parents will show up on your doorstep one day, or that your child will seek them out? Do you feel that your child's biological parents, whether personally known or anonymous, will feel like potential rivals to you?

If you find these issues disturbing, you may find that it is helpful to put your fears in context. The concerns that you as a potential adoptive parent are experiencing all have their counterpart in the kinds of concerns that biological parents face. Thus, your concern that your child's love will be taken away by his biological parents really raises a question all parents must face . . . namely, will my child continue to love me when he's older, or will he reject me? Biology does not create love. Similarly, your worry about what to tell your adoptive child about his origins has its analogue in an issue which all humans must deal with. When one sets out to produce a baby one is dealing with a genetic process that is quite random. There is no way of determining which egg will unite with which sperm, to form a particular embryo, and eventually a particular child. One's genetic history is largely accidental. There is no guarantee that one's child will get your "good" qualities. It might just as easily inherit your less desirable traits or, worse, those of your detested in-laws! If this rationale fails to convince your adoptive child that he is no worse biologically for not coming from you, it should at least dispel another preadoptive parental concern: that an adopted child will not be as "good" as what you could have produced.

Lastly, in assessing whether or not adoption is for you, you must also determine whether you are willing to expend the time, energy, and financial resources it often takes. It is widely acknowledged that obtaining a child for adoption and legalizing an adoption require herculean efforts. This is when your motivation and emotional acceptance of adoption are tested, for it is rare that an adoptable child falls out of the sky and into one's home. Couples must look at alternatives — childlessness, no more children, or a total reliance upon their own reproductive organs. At some point, those who choose adoption simply refuse to be denied or scared off and determine that they will do whatever it takes.

Sometimes the effort required is considerable. As the various means of adopting are explored, decisions must again be made and new fears overcome. Unfortunately, no matter how motivated a couple may be, many are sidetracked for years by a lack of correct information. Because laws, agency rules and sources of babies vary and are all subject to change, the most successful couples leave no stone unturned, scrutinize all sources of information and refuse to accept "no" for an answer.

Part of the decision to adopt a child is the acceptance of the fact that, like producing a child biologically, it is not necessarily going to be easy. It may cost time, energy, and money. It may cause frustration, embarrassment, and sadness. It is good practice for the tough side of parenthood.

Practical questions influence whether and by what means a couple pursues adoption. Some couples are immediately attracted to children who are handicapped, older, part of a group of siblings, and/or not of their race. Other couples want only what they had hoped to produce themselves: a healthy infant of their own general appearance. Some couples prefer an agency-arranged placement because it provides the most legal safeguards from a change of heart by the biological parents during the pendency of the adoption. Other couples may choose private adoption, either because they prefer to know the birth parents as well as possible, or because they were judged ineligible for consideration by the agencies to which they applied. State laws that either allow or forbid private adoption also dictate the course of action a couple can take. The decision to adopt is, then, really a two-step process: first, the decision that adoption is desired must be reached; second, after an investigation of available resources, the method of making it happen has to be determined.

AGENCY ADOPTION

The most common and accepted way in which prospective adoptive parents seek to find a child is through a licensed domestic adoption agency, which acts as a socially approved intermediary whose task it is to distribute a limited supply of children to those who seem to it most suitable.

The average wait for a healthy newborn in the United States is currently somewhere between three and five years. The situation for hard-to-place children — those older than eight years, minority children, children who are part of a sibling group, and children with physical, intellectual, or emotional handicaps — is generally less discouraging. This is because there are more children in these categories available for placement, as well as fewer prospective parents whose first choice is a hard-to-place child. Both the selection criteria that agencies use and the length of time you should expect to wait before being given a child reflect these realities.

In order to make your decision about whether or not you wish to pursue adoption through an agency, it is important to know both some of the advantages and disadvantages of selecting this route.

The primary reason that leads couples to adopt through an agency is that agencies are still the greatest source of children. Equally important to many is the fact that agency adoption affords them the best legal safeguards. Before an agency will place a child in your home, both birth parents are required to sign papers relinquishing the child. This relinquishment is final unless obtained under false pretenses or under duress. Once the child is placed in your home by an agency, you can relax in the knowledge that the parents have forfeited their rights and cannot at any time change their minds about this and successfully seek to reclaim their child. An additional plus is that the agency acts as go-between in the transaction between biological and adoptive parents, thereby assuring anonymity for both. The agency also attempts to investigate both the health and backgrounds of the biological parents and the health of the child it places with you, so that you can be as informed as possible about what difficulties you might encounter. Lastly, agencies locate the babies they place, thereby requiring of the prospective adoptive parents far less initiative than if they were to search for a child on their own.

There are several reasons why agency adoption is not the route taken by all those who seek to adopt. Foremost, agency adoption, particularly of healthy newborns, is highly competitive. The selection criteria that agencies use are designed to select those individuals who they believe will best be able to meet the needs of the child waiting to be adopted. These criteria are set and administered by each individual agency. This means that if they do not see you as meeting their criteria for successful adoptive parents, you will either be discouraged from applying at all, or in less clearcut situations you may be rejected once your application is reviewed. Some of the criteria that agencies use in making their selection will be detailed later.

Some individuals or couples who might be found to be suitable candidates by an agency also choose to look elsewhere for a child. Some feel that the entire application process and home study is an invasion of privacy. Others feel resentful that because they are infertile they have to prove that they would be suitable parents. The long waiting period for a child is still another deterrent, as is the three- to six-month interval between birth and placement of a newborn by an agency that must obtain final relinquishment papers and legalize the surrender before placing a child. Those who prefer to search for a child themselves, and those who feel that they want to get to know the biological mother or parents directly may also find that an agency adoption does not meet their needs.

Finding an Agency

Let us suppose that after weighing the pros and cons you have decided that you would like to adopt through an agency. The first thing that you have to do after making this decision is to find an agency. If you live near a large city there are probably a number of agencies from which to choose. There are two types of agencies: public and private. Public agencies are supported by taxes and run by the city or county department of welfare or social services. Generally, the fees you would be expected to pay are lowest in a public agency. Private agencies can be either nonsectarian or affiliated with and financed by a specific religious group. The latter specializes in adoptions for children and parents of a specific religion: Catholic, Jewish, and so on. Private agencies usually have more funding than do public agencies and thus are able to offer more in the way of counseling services to both biological and adoptive parents. The fees you will be asked to pay are usually somewhat higher at private than at public agencies. However, most agencies do have sliding fee scales based on a percentage of your yearly income.

The first thing you need to do is to find out which agencies are located in your area. Consult your telephone directory under "Adoption Agency," also call or write to your city, county, or state department of social services for information. Adoptive parents groups in your area are another potential source of information, both to help you find out about specific agencies and also to provide you with information about which agencies are taking applications, what different agencies are looking for, what kinds of children each has available, and how best to present yourself to maximize your chances of being placed on their waiting list.

Information about how to locate adoptive parents' groups in your area may be obtained by contacting local agencies or through adoption information services such as the Open Door Society, the North American Council on Adoptable Children, and the newsletter of OURS, Inc. (see Adoption Resources).

In your search for an agency keep in mind that policies and practices of agencies differ widely. In making an initial selection you will want to determine whether or not the agency will consider applicants from your geographic area. Most of them require that you live within a certain distance in order to facilitate home study interviews and court appearances. In addition, you will want to determine if they accept applicants of your religious affiliation and if they place children in the age range you prefer.

The Application Procedure

The first hurdle that you have to master is finding an agency that will put you on their waiting list. Call or write whichever agencies you think may be receptive to you, informing them of your interest. Inquire whether the agency is accepting applications, if they handle children of the age you desire, and whether you would be eligible to apply. Most agencies will not accept applications from couples wishing to adopt an infant if they do not have a fertility problem. Similarly, you may find that an agency may require that prospective parents be between given upper and lower age limits or that they have a requirement that you have been married at least two years before applying. You may also ask about special adoption services for older, minority, and special-needs children, and whether you would be considered for this type of placement. Some agencies will accept applications from couples who know they are fertile or from single individuals only if the applicant is willing to consider taking such a hard-to-place child.

If an agency is not taking applications, ask when they expect to be taking them again. Also ask for information regarding other agencies in your area that are currently accepting applications. They may also be able to tell you which agencies accept applications from fertile couples and single individuals.

Once you have found an agency that is accepting applications, you are ready to embark on the application process. The first step is to meet with the agency individually or with a group of applicants, depending on the policy of the given agency. This initial "information meeting" will be one that the agency uses to acquaint you with their policies and procedures. They will tell you what kinds of children they have available, what kinds of homes they are seeking, and what the anticipated waiting period is. They will also discuss the application process, agency requirements, and fees. You will be given an application form at the close of the meeting if you wish to pursue the application process further.

You will take the application form home with you, and when you have completed it, return it to the agency. Each agency has its own form. However, what is common to all of them is that they provide the agency with an effective screening device. This means that how you deal with this initial application may have a direct bearing on whether or not they will go on to approve you as an adoptive parent. As part of the application you will be asked to provide copies of some standard documents such as birth certificates, your marriage certificate, a divorce decree if either of you has been married and divorced in the past, proof of nationality, a W-2 tax form from the previous year, bank statements, insurance policies, and titles to any real estate that you may own. In addition, you will be asked to supply the agency with basic factual information about both you and your spouse. Some agencies request that each of you also submit an autobiography. It is customary for the agency to ask you to give them several references (somewhere between three and six, depending on the agency). References from your employer, your physician, or your clergyman may also be requested. A medical assessment of both your physical and emotional fitness, as well as your fertility status, will be requested from your physician. You will also be asked to fill out a financial report.

In filling out this application, you will naturally want to present yourselves in the most favorable light possible, in order to maximize your chances of obtaining the child you want. In her informative book *Beating the Adoption Game,* Cynthia Martin, a clinical psychologist with wide experience in all areas of adoption, presents many ideas about how to do this effectively. She advises that since the agency has what you want most, a child, either you tell them what they want to hear or you risk being turned down for not meeting their unstated criteria. For instance, your autobiography should emphasize your strengths, talents, and achievements, as well as those qualities and experiences that will demonstrate to the agency that you have what it takes to be a successful adoptive parent.

Similarly, it is critical that you select as references people who know and like you, and who can vouch for your fitness to raise a child. Before submitting names to the agency it will be worth your while to ask each potential reference whether they feel that they can write a strong letter on your behalf. Remember, this is a highly competitive arena, and a lukewarm letter may put you out of the running.

It is also advisable to be open-minded from the outset. For example, if you state that you want only a healthy white infant, and find the idea of adopting any other type of child unacceptable, most agencies will not even consider taking your application. Since there are few healthy white infants to be placed, agencies want to accept potential parents who are willing to consider adopting children from a wider spectrum. So, in order even to be in the running you might indicate that you are more flexible than you may actually be. Once your application has been accepted, and then approved, you still have the right to turn down any particular child who may be offered to you. Agreeing to consider a range of possibilities makes you eligible to participate in the agency process; it does not obligate you to accept a child you do not want.

The Home Study
Once you have returned your application form to the agency, you will be assigned a social worker, who as a representative of the

agency will be the one to conduct an "adoption" or "home" study. Its purpose is to allow the agency to know you well enough so that they can assess whether, in their opinion, you will be able to meet the needs of the child they place with you. In addition, the home study attempts to help you explore your thoughts and feelings about adoption, as well as your feelings about being an adoptive parent. If you decide that you want to continue to pursue adoption, your worker will use the home study to help prepare you for the adjustments of adoption. A fairly typical home study might consist of three interviews, two conducted at the agency and a third at your home. In addition to these joint interviews with you and your spouse, some agencies also conduct separate interviews with each potential parent.

Although all agencies admit that it is difficult to predict who will and who will not be a successful adoptive parent, each has its own selection criteria. Trying to learn what an agency might look for in prospective adoptive parents, we talked to an adoption worker who has been employed by a private agency for many years. The following is a list of the kinds of attributes that this worker looks for.

1. Emotional Maturity — for example, how well each of you copes with difficulty, uncertainty, and frustration and how you have dealt with life crises.

2. Quality of Relationships with Others — how you relate to others; whether you are able to accept differences in others; whether you have the capacity to adjust and change in your relationships; and if you are capable of warm and loving relationships.

3. Quality of the Marital Relationship — is your marriage stable? Do you and your spouse treat each other with warmth and mutual respect?

4. Feelings toward Children — how much experience have you had with children? What kind of child do you desire, and why? Do you and your spouse each — independently — desire a child?

5. Flexibility — this includes both how flexible you are able to be regarding the type of child you are willing to consider and whether you will be able to be an open and flexible parent.

6. Acceptance of Infertility — have you and your spouse come to terms with your inability to produce a biological child? Do you see adoption as an acceptable alternative way to have a child in your life?

7. Readiness to Adopt — are you aware of the implications of adoption for both you and your child? Are you able to accept the fact that your child will grow up with an extra parent (or two) always in the background, even if never present? Are you prepared to handle the issue of adoption with your child? Are you ready for parenthood? Is the marriage ready for children?

8. Ability to Integrate a Child into Your Family — if you already have biological children, will you be able to love an adopted child as much; will you be able to make him or her part of your family?

9. Single Parenthood — if you are single, are you able to support a child of your own? Can you provide a home for a child? Can you provide a child with a full life, including relationships with men, women, and families? Will a child be an addition to your life, and not a replacement for anything that is missing from it?

10. Health Status — are you physically and emotionally fit to raise a child? Do you have any condition that may interfere with your ability to be a parent, or that might shorten your life? (Most agencies claim that they have no absolute rules as to health requirements for adoptive parents — that each case is reviewed individually.)

11. Financial Stability — is your income adequate to raise a child? (Here, agencies claim to look, not at how much money you make, but rather, how well you manage your financial resources.) Many states are able to provide adoption subsidies. These are awarded primarily to low-income families and to foster parents who wish to adopt. In addition, most sates offer both direct and medical subsidies to parents who adopt children with special needs.

After your home study is completed, your worker will submit the information she has collected to the agency for final consideration. Occasionally prospective adopters are rejected at this point. Some of the reasons that agencies give for rejecting applicants include the presence of marital problems, major medical problems, or personality problems in either parent.

If you are rejected, it is theoretically possible to reapply at a later time; the rejection is not irreversible. Find out why you were rejected. If your caseworker is unwilling to supply you with this information, demand of the agency administration that you be informed. Some couples have enlisted the aid of government officials in their local area, when they were unable to obtain an explanation by other means. Do what you have to in order to find out what you want to know. Once you learn the reason for being turned down, you will want to consider whether there is anything that you can do to reverse the decision. Remember, a rejection does not mean that you are bad or unfit: what it indicates is that you did not meet the agency's criteria for ideal adoptive parents.

Most likely, your application will be approved and you will be placed on the agency's waiting list for a child. As stated earlier, the length of time you will have to wait before a child is placed with you cannot be predicted. A wait of three to five years is about average at the present time for a healthy infant, while the wait for a hard-to-place child will usually be far shorter than this.

After a long or short wait you will enter the pool of applicants that the agency is actively considering. When the agency locates a child that they feel will be suitable for you, your social worker will let you know that there is a child for you to consider. She will share with you information about the child's age, his general appearance, his race and national background, the history of his mother's pregnancy if he is newborn, his medical status, and, if the child is older, his personality traits. You will also be given some information about the child's biological parents: their age, race, religion, physical health, mental health, educational or work background, and information about why they are giving the child up for adoption. If after you learn about the child you are interested in considering him or her, the agency will arrange for you to meet him or her. When placing an older child, the agency usually holds several meetings before final placement is made. This gives both the adoptive parents and the child a chance to see if the placement is acceptable. Sometimes, a trial placement may be suggested.

Placement of the child in your home is usually followed by several more visits by the adoption worker. She will use these to assess how well everyone is adjusting, and to make a final assessment of the appropriateness of the placement. Although the child is in your home, he is not legally your child until the adoption is completed in court. How long after placement you will have to wait to go to court depends on the law in the state in which you live. The required waiting period is not just a pro forma requirement: although agencies rarely reclaim the children they place, they do have a legal right to do so.

In the case of a child older than twelve years, his consent will be required at the court hearing. This is the final step in making your long-awaited child truly yours.

INDEPENDENT, DIRECT, OR PRIVATE ADOPTION

Private adoption (the terms "independent" and "direct" adoption are synonymous with private adoption) and agency adoption can be pursued simultaneously. Therefore, unless a couple has a strong need to meet or know the biological mother (and/or father) of their adoptive child, or an unusually strong aversion to bureaucratic red tape, they can lose nothing by signing up with local agencies.

For couples that are unable to qualify with their local agencies, private adoption is an alternative means to adopting a child. If you do not qualify, it is very important that this setback not be blown up out of proportion. Not qualifying does not in any way mean that you are unfit or incapable of being excellent parents. Rather, it is a reflection of the relative shortage of children available to the particular agency for placement.

In a private adoption the biological parents "place" their child with the adoptive parents "directly," or "independently" of agencies; in an agency adoption, the parents "place" a child with an agency, which, after obtaining custody, then "places" the child with a chosen couple.

In a private adoption, the burden of finding a child who is available for adoption falls on you rather than on a third party.

Private adoption is legal in all but the following states: Colorado, Connecticut, Delaware, Massachusetts, Michigan, and Minnesota. However, make certain that it is legal in *your* state of residence before embarking on your own search for a child to adopt privately.

If your state laws prohibit private adoption, you may want to abandon the idea, or you may want to consider the possibility of moving your residence to a state where private adoption is legal. You should be certain, however, that private adoption really is illegal. For example, in Massachusetts, although private adoption is "illegal," agencies are permitted to "facilitate" private placements through a process known as "identified adoption." There, a couple that knows of a baby available for a potential private placement can come within the law by hiring an agency to perform its usual function with respect to obtaining relinquishments and doing a home study, but treating the placement as a fait accompli.

It is important to find out what the specific legal process for private adoption is in your state. The best source of information on this is likely to be a lawyer who specializes in adoption. Because adoption is not an everyday case for most lawyers, it is best to consult a lawyer who can speak from experience. Couples who have previously adopted a child through private adoption are a particularly good referral source. So too, are other lawyers, doctors, and social workers.

The procedures in private adoption vary greatly because they were created by state law. However, the general concept of private adoption is fairly uniform. Typically, a mother or mother-to-be reaches a decision that she does not have the ability or desire to raise her child. She concludes that adoption will best serve the child's interest, and learns of a couple that is willing and able to provide the child with parents and a loving, stable, permanent home. As soon as possible after birth, the child is physically placed with the adoptive parents, who then petition the court for an adoption decree that will legally create a parent-child relationship between them. After a period of some months (the exact waiting period differs from state to state), and with the benefit of a social service report (prepared by a government social agency) on the family, a judge terminates the biological parent-child relationship and grants the adoption.

In private adoption the final relinquishment papers are not signed until several months after the child is placed in the adoptive home, unlike agency adoption, where the mother has signed away her rights before placement. In a private adoption, then, since the adoption is not legally complete until several months after the child has been placed, the child could be reclaimed by the biological parents if they so wish. While this rarely occurs, it is a possibility and constitutes the single major drawback to private adoption: should the biological parents change their minds, the adoptive parents may have to give the child back. Since the regulations are subject to variations in state law, the applicable rules should be *thoroughly discussed* at the initial legal consultation. The prospect of having to return your child to its biological parents is frightening. It is an excellent reason for doing your best to evaluate the biological parents' certainty *before* the child is placed. Fortunately, "reclamations" or "reversals" are not very common. Although accurate statistics are hard to find, knowledgeable persons working in the adoption field have offered estimates of anywhere from 1 out of 25 to less than 1 in 50. If these figures are even remotely accurate, one's chances of losing a child because of parental change of heart are far less than of losing one during pregnancy. This somewhat grim reality is mentioned, however, as a reminder that getting a child, by whatever method, is risky.

Another aspect of private adoption which often worries prospective adoptive parents is that in private adoption the biological mother and father (if he is known) and the adoptive couple know each other's identities. In practice, the amount of contact between biological and adoptive parents varies greatly. If all parties desire, they may get to know each other reasonably well. Alternatively, a mutual decision may be made to keep contact to a minimum. In the latter situation, a third party, a friend, doctor, lawyer, relative, or other intermediary, may assist the biological mother in finding out what she needs to know about the prospective adoptive parents.

Most couples find that lack of anonymity in private adoption disturbing at first. The usual fear is that, some day in the future, the biological mother will show up in their home or in the schoolyard and create an indescribably painful scene. Our experience has been that this is not the case. In fact, in sharp contrast to everyone's worst fears, meetings between the adoptive and biological parents are almost always very positive experiences. Seeing each other in the flesh can be extremely reassuring to all concerned. The biological parents can see for themselves that the adoptive parents are willing and able to love and care for their child. Similarly, a

first-hand meeting gives the prospective adoptive parents an opportunity to evaluate in person how certain the biological parents
are about their decision to give their child up for adoption.
Usually, the reasons for relinquishing the child make sense, and it
becomes obvious that fears of future harassment were largely fan-
ciful.

Where such direct encounters between natural and adoptive
parents do occur, they serve an additional function: the adoptive
couple will be better able to satisfy the child's curiosity about his or
her birth parents when the time comes to discuss the "facts of life."

Cost

Rumor has it that only wealthy couples, willing to buy a child, can
engage in private adoption. In fact, although both birth-related
expenses and legal fees for the adoption are customarily paid by
the adoptive couple, it is illegal for anyone to profit unduly from
the placement of a child. Black-market adoption, or baby selling, is
not legal in any state.

Before you go ahead with a private adoption it is, however, important to know that, in general, the money you will pay out is
nonrefundable. This means that in the event of a change of heart
by the natural parents, they have no legal obligation to reimburse
you. The reason for this is that the law requires that the parental
consent be completely free and voluntary. An adoptive *placement*
(before the final court appearance) is not a contractual relationship. It is viewed as an *offer* of a home by the prospective adoptive
parents, who knowingly accept the risk involved.

The one way to be sure that costs are legitimate is to make certain that each expense is itemized and documented. Most couples
have little difficulty finding out the going rate for a particular expense, and so are able to avoid being victimized. Only customary,
reasonable fees can be charged.

It is usually possible to get a fairly accurate idea about how
much the adoption will cost before you decide to go through with
it. Costs can vary from as low as $500 to as much as $5,000 or
more. Of course, sometimes unplanned-for expenses do arise, such
as uninsured medical bills that may be higher than anticipated (if,
for example, a cesarean delivery must be performed), or if there are

travel expenses for the mother or mother-to-be to deliver the child to you or for you to pick up the child from her.

Finding a Child to Adopt

How do you go about finding a child to adopt? There is no single answer to this question. Basically, what is necessary is to make contact, no matter how indirectly at first, with a woman who has a child she wishes to place. There are many different ways to accomplish this. Some people work through their doctor, lawyer, or clergyman. Others tell everyone they know that they are looking for a child, in the hope that a wide net will increase their chance of being successful. Generally, it is wise to let as many people as you can know that you are seeking a child to adopt. In addition, you might encourage your contacts to spread the word to everyone that they know. This is one time when you want the human gossip network to work for you. For example, you tell a friend who is a nurse. She tells all her friends and acquaintances, many of whom are also nurses, and so on. Remember, the more people out there who are looking for you, the better your chance of success.

Some people do not confine their search to their own circle of acquaintances or even to their own geographic area. Some write to people they know of all over the country. Blind mailings have been known to produce good leads. Your search can extend as far as the limits of your creativity, your energy, or your financial resources — it all depends on how determined you are.

Since it is impossible to predict where and when a lead will appear, it is necessary that you prepare yourself for instant success before you let the word out. Paul and Joan had this experience. Two weeks after writing a letter to their physician uncle in another state, they received a call from a colleague of his. He informed them that he had a patient who had just delivered a healthy boy and was looking for a couple to adopt the child. After some frantic searching they were able to locate a lawyer who was knowledgeable about private adoption in their state. With the help of their newly found lawyer they were able within a week's time to evaluate the lead that had come their way, follow it up, and arrange for the adoption of their son.

Of course, not everyone is as fortunate as Paul and Joan. Sometimes it takes a lot more searching before a lead is unearthed. Sometimes one that at first looked promising does not work out. It cannot be overemphasized that once a possibility is located it must be carefully evaluated; some are better than others. Before committing yourself emotionally or financially, you should obtain as much information as possible. Areas that it is important to find out about include the certainty of the birth parents' decision to relinquish the child, the parents' health, and if the child is already born, his or her health, estimated costs, and any potential legal problems that may exist.

It is important that you feel good about a lead before getting too deeply involved. Acting out of a sense of desperation is a greater mistake than being too choosy. There will be other possibilities, and it is a bad idea to go against one's better judgment.

It is also a good idea to be ready for something to go wrong. Leads have been known to fizzle before a placement occurs. The decision to give away one's child is a difficult one for most people. Frequently, especially around the time of the birth, there is a change of heart by the biological parent or parents. The couple that holds back emotionally until the actual placement occurs is best able to cope with these "adoptive miscarriages" and to get ready for the next possibility.

The Placement

Assuming all goes well, the actual placement usually takes place as soon as possible. With newborns, if the biological parent agrees, the adoptive couple can even take care of the baby in the nursery. At the birth parents' option, they can sign the child out of the hospital to the adoptive parents or make the transfer personally outside.

Once the child is placed in the adoptive home, the legal petition for adoption is filed. Thereafter, a state social agency does an investigation and makes a report, which is filed with the court. The report usually contains a recommendation that the adoption be granted and gives background information. The information, which was gathered by the adoption worker, usually includes biographical facts about the adoptive couple and biological parents, medical information, references, and other relevant data.

Finally, when the report has been filed, the consents of the biological parents have been taken, and the statutory time period of waiting (if any) has gone by, the adoption is completed in court.

The court appearance is usually only a formality and lasts only a few minutes. Judges tend to give solemn advice or make friendly jokes before sending the happy parents on their way. One couple was told by the judge, "I adopted a child myself. We figured we needed some brains and good looks in the family."

INTERCOUNTRY ADOPTION

In an intercountry, or international, adoption, you, the adoptive parent, adopt a child born in another country. The adoption is legalized either in the country of the child's birth or in your state of residence in the United States (depending on various factors, including your state's laws and the laws of the particular foreign country).

Is Intercountry Adoption a Possibility for You?

If you've made the decision to adopt a child, if you have positive feelings about becoming a transracial/transcultural family forever, if you can accept the unknowns in the life of a foreign-born child, if you have the patience, energy, flexibility, and determination to deal with the complexities of intercountry adoption, if you have the financial resources to meet the costs of intercountry adoption — then intercountry adoption could be an option for you in building a family through adoption.

In educating yourself about intercountry adoption, you'll find out about the need for racial and cultural awareness if your family is to become transracial and transcultural. You'll read and hear about the benefits of learning about your child's heritage — about racial and cultural origins — and about teaching the whole family as your child grows. It's an exciting and stimulating process.

Who Chooses Intercountry Adoption?

People who choose intercountry adoption are often couples who would qualify for domestic agency adoption of a healthy infant but who don't want to wait five years or longer, couples (or single persons) who are rejected by local agencies for domestic infant adoption for a variety of reasons (for example, their age or having two or more children at home already — even if these are children from a previous marriage — or being single), and people who actively seek to adopt foreign-born special-needs children: school-age children, sibling groups, physically and/or mentally challenged children.

The Children

The children available for international adoption come from countries with widespread poverty, countries perhaps suffering the turmoil of war or natural disasters, countries that cannot, at present, provide for their homeless children, countries that look favorably on placing children for adoption internationally, countries where adoption is not an accepted cultural practice, where biological family ties are intensely strong, where an impoverished family cannot feed all of its children, where the unwed mother and the illegitimate child are social outcasts, where there is no bright future for the abandoned or orphaned child — where if the child indeed survives infancy and early childhood, he may grow up in an orphanage, in a hospital, in a prison, or simply in the streets.

In 1981, United States citizens were adopting children almost exclusively from Asia (Korea, Japan, Thailand, Hong Kong, Taiwan, the Philippines, India) and from Latin America (almost all countries of Central and South America). In some of these countries, there are many children who can be legally freed for adoption, and the process of international adoption is straightforward and fairly routine; in other countries, there are very few children actually available for international adoption and the procedures may be quite complicated and/or time-consuming.

Babies are usually available through international adoption agencies as well as through private contacts. At times, your wait for an infant could be much longer (many months, even two years or longer) than the wait for a preschool or school-age child, a sibling group, or a handicapped child. At other times, the offer of an infant might come within a few months after you've been accepted by your foreign contact or by the United States–based agency helping you with your adoption.

As part of the home study and application process, you'll consider the age range that you'd be able to accept, being as flexible as possible, yet honest about your feelings. Be aware, too, that babies and older children with correctable medical problems (cleft palate, for instance) are often considered hard to place and are therefore readily available for adoption.

Where Do You Start?

"Put as many irons in the fire as you can": . . . valuable advice for prospective adoptive parents who are pursuing *any* kind of adoption. What exactly does this mean for you if you are interested in intercountry adoption? First, it's always helpful to tell as many people as you can that you are planning to adopt and that you are interested in intercountry adoption. This increases your chances of (1) hearing about new developments: for example, new agencies, new sources of children; (2) being given personal contacts in foreign countries; (3) learning about individual families and/or adoptive parents' groups in your area who've had experience in intercountry adoption and would gladly share knowledge and give you the opportunity to meet their children.

You might begin cautiously by attending an information meeting offered by an adoption agency or an adoptive parents' group; by reading materials on intercountry adoption, transracial adoption, and the countries involved in intercountry adoption; by talking to people who've adopted internationally and meeting their children. You might even find a course for prospective adoptive parents taught at a local college. NOTE: It doesn't hurt — and costs so little — to do all these things at once even as you develop your thoughts about adopting, confirm your desires, and gather information on *all* possible sources for a child.

The best place to start is with an adoptive parents' support group that has members who are knowledgeable about intercountry adoptions. Your contact can acquaint you with state and federal regulations affecting intercountry adoption; with the countries most likely to be placing children for international adoption with United States citizens; with your local sources (agency or private social worker) for a home study (federal law requires a home study for all intercountry adoptions). The parents' group can also give you up-to-date information about United States–based international adoption agencies and possibly about foreign contacts for parent-initiated adoptions.

Types of Intercountry Adoption

There are two types of intercountry adoption: agency (agency-to-agency) adoptions and parent-initiated adoptions. In the former, a United States adoption agency has made child-placing agreements with a foreign agency or with a United States–based international adoption agency. For the prospective adoptive parents, most of the paperwork involved in this process is taken care of by the agencies. After your applications have been accepted and your home study has been approved, a child is selected and offered to you (all of these steps involve time and [im]patient waiting!). You can expect to receive a photograph of the child you are considering as well as his or her medical and social histories. Often, once a placement is made, the child is escorted to the United States, though sometimes parents must travel to the child's country in order to bring him or her home.

In parent-initiated adoptions, the prospective adoptive parents must, for the most part, arrange the adoption themselves: that is, you as the adopter find the foreign source willing to accept your application for a child; you obtain a home study; you are personally responsible for sending official translations of all documents to the proper authorities of the country where you're planning to adopt; you communicate directly with your foreign contact (keeping the local social worker informed) and with the foreign attorney; you work directly with the United States Immigration Service to obtain an entry visa for your child; and you travel to your child's country to escort the child home.

The language barrier and the lack of personal or face-to-face contact with your source may pose risks or present complications that are usually avoidable with agency adoptions. On the other hand, some people view these factors merely as a challenge.

Costs

Intercountry adoption is not an inexpensive way to adopt a child. Costs range from $2,000 to $4,500 or more. Fees you should expect to pay in any intercountry adoption are your local home study fee (these vary greatly), an immigration fee for your child's visa, and air fare for you and/or your child. In addition, you may pay a fee to the foreign agency placing your child; a fee to a liaison agency helping in the placement; translation fees; notarization, verification, and authentication fees. You may want to make a donation to the organization that cared for your child before the adoption (an orphanage, for example), and you may want to send or take supplies needed in caring for infants and children.

Advice from Those Who Chose Intercountry Adoption: The Process Is Often Hard Work, but the Results Are Worth It!!
It's important to bear in mind that the adoption picture could change at any time in a particular country (and that new state or federal laws enacted in the United States *or* new interpretations of existing regulations could affect your intercountry adoption as well). For example, political unrest and a change of government can dramatically and suddenly alter the adoption situation. This is where your ability to be flexible and patient is essential.

Realize that you'll need fortitude, patience, optimism, and determination in pursuing intercountry adoption. For an agency-assisted intercountry adoption, you'll probably needs lots of patience and fortitude; for a parent-initiated intercountry adoption, you'll need a great deal of energy and determination. You'll *always* need optimism — and that can be bolstered by seeking the reassuring support of other adoptive parents and by reading everything you can in the adoption literature. Of course, your determination and creative energy in pursuing intercountry adoption will still be the key to finding your child.

Acknowledgments

Surviving Pregnancy Loss is the product of many people's efforts. We are grateful to all who talked with us, filled out our lengthy questionnaire, shared their experiences, and often, despite their own pain, helped and encouraged us along the way.

Special thanks to the following people for contributing a detailed account of their personal experiences: Craig Anderson for "The Husband's Experience"; Judith Wrubel for "Ectopic Pregnancy: One Woman's Experience"; Margaret S. Ross, M.D., for "Miscarriage: One Woman's Experience"; and Charlene Arcidiacono for "Stillbirth: One Woman's Experience." We are indebted to each of you for sharing so much, your hopes and fears, your pain and disappointment, your words of advice and your spirit to survive.

Our warm thanks also to the friends and colleagues whose generous contributions we warmly appreciate: Tate Snyder for "Intercountry Adoption"; Darlene Peck, R.N., for sharing her work on the role of the health care professional; Sal Lopes for sharing his thoughts about how men experience the loss of a pregnancy; Lora Tessman, Ph.D., Lois Eichler, Ph.D., and Miriam Mazor, M.D., for many germinative conversations; Karen Cohen for coleading the original miscarriage support group and for collaborating on subsequent projects; Robert H. Friedman, M.D., for his help and support throughout; Marc Gradstein, attorney-at-law, for serving as consultant on legal issues and for his contribution to the private adoption chapter; Mary Tondorf-Dick, our thoughtful and sensitive editor, who shared our vision and helped it take form; and Barbara Eck Menning, R.N., for her pioneering work in the field and for her excellent foreword.

Thanks also go to Bette Greene, Alaina Anderson, Lee Dauber, Hannah Hecht, Stephanie Blumberg, Cecile Terrien Lampton and David Lampton, Susan Laughlin, D.S.W., Alexis Aquino Mackles, Annelise Rothman, Linda Ataide, R.N., Donna Benedict, R.N., Jane Butler, R.N., Lowell Cooper, Ph.D., Philip J. Hoffman, M.D., Russell K. Laros, M.D., Lawrence Mackles, M.D., Peter McConarty, M.D., and Davis S. Chapin, M.D.

We would like to thank The Compassionate Friends, Resolve, Inc., and Sister Jane Marie Lamb, SHARE Chairperson, for assisting us in collecting the information about support organizations.

We also would like to thank Kathy Gossett, Eileen Cox, Jordana Friedman, Sharon Pellegrino, and Julie S. Roberts for their help with the manuscript.

We are deeply indebted to Robert Glass, M.D., who offered continual encouragement and advice throughout the writing of this book, generously gave of his time to write a foreword, shared his expertise on the medical aspects of pregnancy loss, and served as a sounding board through the years of researching and writing this book.

Appendix: Resources

National Support Organizations

This information was obtained in 1981. Since groups disband, leaders change, and people move, the reader is advised that some entries may not continue to be correct.

AMEND (Aiding a Mother Experiencing Neonatal Death)
National Headquarters: Mrs. Maureen Connelly, 4324 Berrywick Terrace, St. Louis, MO 63128. (314) 487-7582.
A service of The Life Seekers. Volunteer counselors offer support and encouragement to parents who have experienced a neonatal death.

The Compassionate Friends
National Headquarters: P.O. Box 1347, Oak Brook, IL 60521. (312) 323-5010.
Self-help organization for parents who have lost a child. Approximately 270 chapters in the United States and worldwide.

National Sudden Infant Death Syndrome Foundation
Two Metro Plaza, Suite 205, 8240 Professional Place, Landover, MD 20785.
Provides public information about SIDS and aid to families who have experienced a sudden infant death.

Resolve, Inc.
National Headquarters: P.O. Box 474, Belmont, MA 02178. (617) 484-2424.
Branches in 35 cities, 12 additional branches in process of organizing. Support organization for those who have experienced infertility or pregnancy loss.

SHARE (A Source of Help in Airing and Resolving Experiences)
National Headquarters: St. John's Hospital, 800 East Carpenter Street, Springfield, IL 62702. (217) 544-6464. Sister Jane Marie Lamb, Director.
National networked self-help groups offering support to bereaved parents of newborns.

Local Organizations

ALABAMA
Compassionate Friends–Alabama
Chapters in Birmingham, Huntsville, Montgomery.
Contact National Headquarters for more information.

ARIZONA
Compassionate Friends–Arizona
Chapter in Phoenix.
Contact National Headquarters for more information.

CALIFORNIA
AMEND — California
Chapters in Calabassas/Los Angeles, Harbor City.
Contact National Headquarters for more information.

Compassionate Friends–California
Chapters in Fresno, Hayward/San Francisco, Los Altos/San Francisco, Los Angeles/Lawndale, Los Angeles/Reseda, San Rafael, Ventura.
Contact National Headquarters for more information.

HAND (Helping After Neonatal Death)
P.O. Box 62, San Anselmo, CA 94960. (415) 459-1770.
Meetings third Wednesday of every month at 7:30 Marin General Hospital, Archives Building. Volunteer group of mothers who have experienced the loss of a baby before, during, or after birth. Offer individual visits, group meetings, sharing of information with helping professionals, contact with sensitive labor coaches trained to assist mothers who are anticipating a stillbirth, volunteer training program, and resource library.
Contact Person: Lisa Jones, 4382 Ranchero Drive, Soquel, CA 95073. (408) 475-4188.

Resolve, Inc.–California
Chapters in Northern California, Orange County.
Contact National Headquarters for more information.

SHARE
Diane Bremseth, 436 Loverne Avenue, Clovis, CA 93612. (209) 299-0008.
This group is affiliated with St. Agnes Hospital in Fresno.

Sharing Parents, A Share Group
Christina Hom, 24 Southlite Circle, Sacramento, CA 95831. (916) 392-7925.

COLORADO

Compassionate Friends–Colorado
Chapters in Colorado Springs, Fort Collins.
Contact National Headquarters for more information.

Newborn and Fetal Loss Support Group, Coordinated by the Parent Education Program
Rose Medical Center, 4567 East Ninth Avenue, Denver, CO 80220. (303) 320-2713.
   Support group, professionally led. Meets twice a month. A community service for anyone in the community who has lost a baby. Funded through the March of Dimes.

Resolve, Inc.–Colorado
Chapters in Denver, Littleton.
Contact National Headquarters for more information.

CONNECTICUT

AID (Aid in Infant Death)
c/o Nancy Baranowski, 28 Wesley Drive, Huntington, CT 06484.
   Support group for parents who have lost babies. Provides hospital visitors, telephone counselors, monthly meetings, pamphlet handed out in local hospitals.

Compassionate Friends–Connecticut
Chapters in Bridgeport, Groton, Stamford.
Contact National Headquarters for more information.

DISTRICT OF COLUMBIA

Resolve, Inc.–Washington, DC
Chapters in Washington Metropolitan area.
Contact National Headquarters for more information.

FLORIDA

AMEND
Karen Frazier, 5104 127th Avenue, Tampa, Florida 33617. (813) 988-7996.

Compassionate Friends–Florida
Chapters in Clearwater, Miami, Miami/Ft. Lauderdale, Orange Park, Orlando, St. Augustine, Sarasota, Tallahassee, Tampa, Titusville, West Palm Beach.
Contact National Headquarters for more information.

Resolve, Inc.–Florida
Chapters in Ft. Lauderdale, Sunrise, Tampa
Contact National Headquarters for more information.

GEORGIA

Compassionate Friends–Georgia
Chapter in Atlanta.
Contact National Headquarters for more information.

Resolve, Inc.–Georgia
Chapter in Atlanta.
Contact National Headquarters for more information.

HAWAII

Compassionate Friends–Hawaii
Chapter in Kahului.
Contact National Headquarters for more information.

ILLINOIS

AMEND
c/o Jane Borman, 2209 Gillis Street, Alton, IL 62002. (618) 466-7129.
Counsels parents who have experienced a newborn death, miscarriage, or stillbirth, on a one-to-one basis. Also provides community education, talks to groups of interested professionals, and a referral service.

Bereaved Parents Group of the Parents and Child Education Society
Contact Person: Cathy McMeilly, 619 S. Humphrey, Oak Park, IL 60304. (312) 848-6154.
Counseling for new parents. Also support services for bereaved parents. Crisis phone line, monthly meetings.

Caretakers
Contact Person: Rev. Robert L. Hansen, Director of Pastoral Care, West Suburban Hospital, 518 North Austin Boulevard, Oak Park, IL 60302. (312) 383-6200 Ext. 6400.
Group for parents who have lost a child during pregnancy or shortly after birth. Open-ended group discussions, films, guest speakers.

Compassionate Friends–Illinois
Chapters in Alton/Moro, Arlington Heights, Aurora, Champaign, Chicago, Hinsdale, Joliet, Lansing, Mattoon, Melrose Park, Oak Forest, Pekin, Rockford, Springfield, Waukegan.
Contact National Headquarters for more information.

ILAC (I Lost A Child)
Contact Persons: Malinda Sawyer, Rt. #5, Box 353, Marion, IL 62959. (618) 997-5233. Jane Hamlin, R.N., Carbondale Memorial Hospital, 404 West Main Street, Carbondale, IL 62901. (618) 549-6735.
Mutual support group for parents who have lost a baby through miscarriage, stillbirth, or infant death.

Loyola Premature High Risk Infant Parents Association
1021 Garner, Wheaton, IL 60187. (312) 852-1910.
A support group for parents of infants in the Loyola Hospital Neo-Natal Unit.

Parents of SIDS
Dr. Goldberg, Medical Coordinator, Loyola Medical Center, 2160 South First Avenue, Maywood, IL 60153. (312) 531-3210.
Monthly meetings at SIDS Regional Center at Loyola.

PACES (Parent and Childbirth Education Society)
P.O. Box 213, Western Springs, IL 60558. (312) 346-5502. Contact Person: Susan Gittings, (312) 848-1630.
Provides people with names of other people in similar circumstances. Provides referrals to other support groups.

Resolve, Inc.–Illinois
Chapter in Chicago.
Contact National Headquarters for more information.

SHARE (Source of Help in Airing and Resolving Experiences)
National Headquarters: St. John's Hospital, 800 East Carpenter Street, Springfield, IL 62702. (217) 544-6464. Sister Jane Marie Lamb, Director. Chapters in Belleville/St. Louis, Champaign/Urbana, Effingham, Jewett, Litchfield, Newton, Pekin, Quincy, Rockford, Vandalia.
Contact National Headquarters for more information.

INDIANA

The Bereaved Parents Group, Sponsored by Parents and Friends of Children of Lincoln Hills, Inc.
c/o Linda K. Runden, A.C.S.W., 101 South Capitol Avenue, Corydon, IN 47112. (812) 738-3277.
Meetings fourth Tuesday of every month except December, at 7 P.M. in University Center Building, Room 009, Indiana University, S.E., West Albany, Indiana. Telephone outreach and support, support group for parents who have lost a child at any time between pregnancy and adolescence. Also groups for sibs and friends.

Bereaved Parents Group
Mrs. William Bear, 2329 Hargan Drive, Madison, IN 47250. Home: (812) 273-1173. Work: (812) 265-2946.

Compassionate Friends–Indiana
Chapters in Anderson, Carmel/Indianapolis, Columbus, Elkhart, Evansville, Fort Wayne, Greenwood, Logansport, Moores Hill, South Bend, Valparaiso, Vincennes.
Contact National Headquarters for more information.

Neo-Fight, Inc.
40 North Ridgeview Drive, Indianapolis, IN 46226. Contact Person: Maureen Greer.
Support group for parents who have had problem pregnancies, stillbirth, infant death, or infants in need of special care. Provides telephone hotline, trained mother to help parents who have an infant in the special care nursery.

Project Comfort
c/o Gerald C. Machgan, Chaplain, Parkview Hospital, 2200 Randalia Drive, Fr. Wayne, IN 46805. (219) 484-6636.
Volunteer staffed group ministering to needs of grieving families who have experienced prenatal losses, or lost a newborn or an infant.

Resolve, Inc.–Indiana
Chapters in Columbus area, Fort Wayne area, Indianapolis area, South Bend.
Contact National Headquarters for more information.

SHARE
Julie Sims, 659 N. 7th Street, Lafayette, IN 47901. (317) 742-6574.

IOWA

Bereaved Parent Group, Parent Share and Support, Inc. (PSAS)
Palmer Memorial Hospital, 112 Jefferson Street, West Union, IA 52175. (319) 422-3811.
Support group for parents who have lost a child of any age.

Compassionate Friends–Iowa
Chapters in Des Moines, Waterloo/Cedar Falls.
Contact National Headquarters for more information.

Resolve, Inc.–Iowa
Chapter in Davenport.
Contact National Headquarters for more information.

Parent to Parent, Part of Parent Share and Support, Inc. (PSAS)
Palmer Memorial Hospital, 112 Jefferson Street, West Union, IA 52175. (319) 422-3811.
Parent-to-parent support after normal birth, stillbirth, neonatal death, or birth of a handicapped child.

SHARE
Debbie Walz, Burlington Medical Center, 602 N. Third, Burlington, IA 62601. (319) 753-3011.

Support Group for Parents with Empty Arms
c/o Dr. Russell C. Striffler, Director of Chaplaincy, St. Luke's Methodist Hospital, 1026 A Avenue, N.E., Cedar Rapids, IA 52407. (319) 369-7347.
Group for parents who have experienced the loss of a baby through miscarriage, stillbirth, premature or unexpected death.

KANSAS

Compassionate Friends–Kansas
Chapters in Kansas City, Topeka.
Contact National Headquarters for more information.

KENTUCKY

Bereaved Parents Group
Rev. Wayne Willis, Norton-Children's Hospitals, Inc., P.O. Box 35070, Louisville, KY 40232.
For those who have lost children older than infants. Monthly meetings.

Compassionate Family (Northern Kentucky)
Contact Persons: Mary Miller, 24 St. Jude Circle, Florence, KY 41042. Rev. Mike Milliken, Grace Episcopal Church, Price Pike, Florence, KY 41042.
For anyone who's experienced the death of a loved one. Meets first Monday of every month at 10:00 A.M. or last Monday of every month at 7:00 P.M.

Compassionate Friends–Kentucky
Chapters in Henderson, Lexington, Louisville, Owensboro.
Contact National Headquarters for more information.

Consoling Parents
c/o Rev. Wayne Willis, P.O. Box 35070, Kosair-Children's Hospital, Louisville, KY 40232. (502) 589-8176.
Monthly meetings, support groups, hotline, referral of bereaved parents to group members through several area hospitals.

For Parents of Children Who Have Died of Sudden Infant Death Syndrome (SIDS).
Contact Persons: Marylou Zesterman, 701 W. North Bend Rd., Cincinnati, OH 45224. (513) 761-9724. Mary Jo Galbaugh, 4185 Boxwood Lane, Independence, KY 41051.

SHARE
Dorothy Van Sant, St. Anthony Hospital, Louisville, KY 40204.

MAINE

Resolve, Inc.–Maine
Chapters in Freeport, Portland.
Contact National Headquarters for more information.

MARYLAND

Compassionate Friends–Maryland
Chapters in Baltimore, Saint Leonard, Wheaton.
Contact National Headquarters for more information.

National Sudden Infant Death Syndrome Foundation
Two Metro Plaza, Suite 205, 8240 Professional Place, Landover, MD 20785.
Provides public information and help to families who have experienced a sudden infant death.

Resolve, Inc.–Maryland
Chapter in Baltimore.
Contact National Headquarters for more information.

MASSACHUSETTS

BACE (Boston Association for Childbirth Education)
Box 29, Newtonville, Mass. 02160.

Boston Stillborn Study Group
Ann Ross, M.S.W., Jean Stringham, A.C.S.W., Judith Riley, A.C.S.W., c/o
Ross, 53 Country Corners Rd., Wayland, MA 01778.
Provides in-service education to hospital staff; talks to interested groups; consultations to professionals; evaluation and treatment of individuals and couples.

Childbirth Education Association of Central Massachusetts, Inc.
c/o Marilyn Bambauer and Linda Brink, P.O. Box 193, West Side Station,
Worcester, MA 01620. (617) 835-2130. (617) 752-0038.
Group for parents experiencing miscarriage, stillbirth, or infant death. Monthly meetings. Also provides lecture and referrals.

Compassionate Friends–Massachusetts
Chapters in Hingham/South Shore, Needham/Boston, North Reading/North Shore, Springfield, South Dennis, Worcester.
Contact National Headquarters for more information.

COPE (Coping with the Overall Pregnancy/Parenting Experience)
Isabel Freeman, M.S.W. Clinical Director, 37 Clarendon Street, Boston, MA
02116. (617) 357-5588.
Provides individual support to women who have had miscarriage or stillbirth. COPE groups and programs are found in 20 Massachusetts communities.

C/SEC (Cesareans/Support, Education and Concern)
15 Maynard Road, Dedham, MA 02026.

HOPE (Help Other Parents Endure)
Contact Person: Sue Harrington, R.N., South Shore Hospital, 55 Fogg Road, South Weymouth, MA 02190. (617) 337-7011, Ext. 332.
Parents' support group, meets second Wednesday of month, 7:30 P.M., Cafeteria.

HOPE (Help Other Parents Endure)
Social Service Department, Winchester Hospital, 41 Highland Avenue, Winchester, MA 01890. (617) 729-9000.
Peer support groups for parents who have lost a child through stillbirth or neonatal death. Monthly meetings.

Massachusetts Regional Center for Sudden Infant Death
Boston City Hospital, 818 Harrison Avenue, Boston, MA 02118. (617) 424-5000.
An organization of parents and professionals who help families learn about and deal with Sudden Infant Death Syndrome.

Neonatal Death Group
Emerson Hospital, Concord, MA 01742. Contact Person: Jill Thibeau, (617) 448-2598.
Self-help group for people who have experienced a miscarriage, stillbirth, or neonatal death. Meets third Wednesday of each month 7:30–9:30 P.M., Cuming Conference Room, Emerson Hospital.

Parents Group, Brigham & Women's Hospital
75 Francis St., Boston, MA 02115, Contact Person: Laura S. Cohen, (617) 732-6462.
Late miscarriage, stillbirth, and neonatal death.

Perinatal Program
Greater Lynn Community Mental Health Center, Union Hospital, 500 Lynnfield Street, Lynn, MA 01940. Coordinator: Barbara Wolf, (617) 598-8800, ext. 501.
Support groups for women who have had a miscarriage or stillbirth.

Resolve, Inc.
National Headquarters: P.O. Box 474, Belmont, MA 02178. (617) 484-2424.

MICHIGAN

Bereaved Parents Group
Contact Person: Mrs. Betty Rabaut, St. Bede's School, 18300 West Twelve Mile Road, Southfield, MI 48076. (313) 559-0578.
Support group for parents who have lost a pregnancy or a child of any age.

Bereaved Parents of Stillborns
Contact Person: Sister Phyllis Sikora, O.P., Chaplain, Providence Hospital,
16001 West Nine Mile Road, Southfield, MI 48075. (313) 424-3000.
*Support group for parents who have experienced the death of a child by stillbirth, mis-
carriage, or neonatal death.*

Compassionate Friends–Michigan
Chapters in Ann Arbor, Benton Harbor, Big Rapids, Detroit, Grand Rapids,
Jackson, Lansing, Traverse City.
Contact National Headquarters for more information.

HOPING (Helping Other Parents In Natural Grief)
Medical Social Work Dept., Edward W. Sparrow Hospital Association, 1215
E. Michigan Avenue, Lansing, MI 48909. (517) 483-2385. Contact Person:
Jeanie Cain, President-Elect, 917 Kenwood, Lansing, MI 48910. (517) 371-
1967.
*Support group made up of parents who have experienced a miscarriage, stillbirth, or the
death of an infant. Offers parent-to-parent support; hospital in-service training, borrow-
ing library, monthly meetings. Meets fourth Thursday of every month in third floor Vol-
unteers Room of Sparrow Hospital's South Annex at 7:30 P.M.*
Contact Person: Mrs. Rosaline Brown, 712 Bush St., Linden, MI 48451. (313)
238-1936.
*Provides one-to-one support that parents need when a child dies (prenatal to one year
after birth).*

PEND (Parents Experiencing Neonatal Death)
Contact Person: Marcia Eager. c/o Neonatal I.C.U., Butterworth Hospital,
100 Michigan Avenue, N.E., Grand Rapids, MI 49503. (616) 774-1774.
*Parent support group — monthly meetings led by Dr. John Khawam, a neonatologist, a
social worker, and a nurse; telephone support. Open to all people in Grand Rapids area.*

Resolve, Inc.–Michigan
Chapter in Ann Arbor.
Contact National Headquarters for more information.

MINNESOTA

Compassionate Friends–Minnesota
Chapters in Detroit Lakes, St. Cloud, Willmar.
Contact National Headquarters for more information.

Resolve, Inc.–Minnesota
Chapter in Twin Cities area.
Contact National Headquarters for more information.

Parents Grief Support Group
Contact Persons: Kathy Peterson and Barbara Elliot, St. Mary's Hospital, Duluth, MN 55805. (218) 726-4000.
Parent support group for people who have experienced miscarriage, stillbirth, or the loss of a child of up to 2 years, including SIDS. Meet second Tuesday each month.

MISSOURI

AMEND (Aiding a Mother Experiencing Neo-Natal Death).
Service offered by the Life Seekers
National Headquarters: Contact Persons: Mrs. Maureen Connelly, 4324 Berrywick Terrace, St. Louis, MO 63128. (314) 487-7582. Mrs. Colleen Nemanick, 12664 Villa Hill, St. Louis, MO 63141.
Peggy Springer, P.O. Box 174, Columbia, MO 65201.
Offers one-to-one counseling to parents who have experienced a stillbirth or a neo-natal death; community education.

Compassionate Friends–Missouri
Chapters in Joplin, Kansas City, St. Louis.
Contact National Headquarters for more information.

HOPE (Helping Other Parents Endure)
Contact Person: Laura Evans, 22 Brixworth, Florissant, MO 63033.
Six-session educational program moderated by professionals for grieving parents.

ESP (Emotional Support for Parents)
Contact Persons: Nancy Watrous and Christine Trampel, 2410 North Garth Avenue, Columbia, MO 65202. (314) 449-3527.
Group of parents within Neo-Fight organization. Offers support to parents experiencing death of a child or crisis involving pregnancy, such as premature delivery, critical neonatal illness, congenital anomalies, Down's syndrome, miscarriage, stillbirth, neonatal death, SIDS, etc.

Mothers-in-Crisis
c/o Terry Weston, Social Service Department, Freeman Hospital, 1102 West 32nd Street, Joplin, MO 64801. (417) 623-2801.
Parent support group: premature, miscarriage, stillbirth, SIDS, and infants who die after birth.

Resolve, Inc.–Missouri
Chapter in St. Louis.
Contact National Headquarters for more information.

SHARE
Contact: Pastoral Care, St. Elizabeth's Hospital, 211 South 3rd Street, Belleville, IL 62221. (618) 234-2120.
Serves greater St. Louis area.

MONTANA

Compassionate Friends–Montana
Chapters in Billings, Eureka, Kalispell.
Contact National Headquarters for more information.

NEBRASKA

Compassionate Friends–Nebraska
Chapters in Chadron, Omaha, Scottsbluff.
Contact National Headquarters for more information.

Resolve, Inc.–Nebraska
Chapter in Lincoln.
Contact National Headquarters for more information.

Wee Care
Contact Person: Philip Gesseling, M.D., Good Samaritan Hospital, Neonatal
Intensive Care Unit, Kearney, NE. (308) 236-4541.
*Support group for parents of children with neonatal difficulties, including neonatal
death.*

NEVADA

Compassionate Friends–Nevada
Chapter in Las Vegas.
Contact National Headquarters for more information.

NEW HAMPSHIRE

Resolve, Inc.–New Hampshire
Chapter in Nashua.
Contact National Headquarters for more information.

NEW JERSEY

Compassionate Friends–New Jersey
Chapters in Audubon, Holmdel, Morristown, Princeton, South Amboy,
South Plainfield, Teaneck, Toms River, Verona.
Contact National Headquarters for more information.

HELP (Helping Endure Loss in Parenthood)
c/o Eileen Thompson, 607 North Oxford Avenue, Ventnor, NJ 08406. (609)
822-5265.
*Support group for parents who have a child dying or who have experienced miscarriage,
stillbirth, early infant death, or the death of an older child. Meetings take place at Shore
Memorial Hospital, Somers Point.*

Resolve, Inc.–New Jersey
Chapters in central New Jersey, northern New Jersey.
Contact National Headquarters for more information.

NEW MEXICO

Compassionate Friends–New Mexico
Chapter in Gallup.
Contact National Headquarters for more information

Resolve, Inc.–New Mexico
Chapter in Albuquerque.
Contact National Headquarters for more information.

NEW YORK

Bereavement and Loss Center of New York
Contact Persons: Anne Rosberger, C.S.W., Executive Director; Henry Rosberger, M.D., Medical Director, 170 E. 83 Street, New York, NY 10028. (212) 879-5655.
Individual, group help.

Bereavement Clinic
c/o Joanne Middleton, Downstate Medical Center, 450 Clarkson Avenue, Brooklyn, NY 11203. (212) 270-1885.
Provides crisis intervention, counseling for parents who have had a miscarriage, still-birth, or neonatal death. Efforts to start parent self-help group are underway.

Compassionate Friends–New York
Chapters in Buffalo, Commack, Delmar/Albany, Geneseo/Naples, New York City, Purdy Station, Rochester, Star Lake.
Contact National Headquarters for more information.

Miscarriage and Stillbirth Support Group
c/o Dorothy Hai, 209 York Street, Olean, NY 14760. (716) 375-2111.
Parent support group. Monthly meetings.

Perinatal Bereavement Council
Contact Persons: Mary and John Wasacz, 172 Madison Road, Scarsdale, NY 10583. (914) 472-5766.
Provides group and one-to-one counseling for parents who have experienced a miscarriage, stillbirth, or early neonatal death.

Resolve, Inc.–New York
Chapters in Albany, Ithaca, Long Island, New York City, Rochester.
Contact National Headquarters for more information.

St. Mary's Bereavement Ministry
Contact Person: Mrs. Carol Carney, East Islip, NY 11730. (516) 277-4759.
Peer counseling for perinatal bereavement, miscarriage, stillbirth, and neonatal death.

St. Philip's Bereavement Ministry
Contact Person: Cindy Pinto, Northport, NY 11768. (516) 261-0495.

SHARE–Syracuse Group
Contact Person: Lois Sugarman, 6726 Gleason Place, Fayetteville, NY 13066.
(315) 446-1262.

NORTH CAROLINA

Compassionate Friends–North Carolina
Chapter in Hickory.
Contact National Headquarters for more information.

Kinder–Mourn
605 East Boulevard, Charlotte, NC 28203. (704) 376-2580 (24-hour call-in
service).
Individual and group support.

NORTH DAKOTA

Compassionate Friends–North Dakota
Chapters in Bismarck, Grand Forks.
Contact National Headquarters for more information.

OHIO

Bereaved Parents Support Group,
Childbirth Education Association of Akron
Contact Persons: Denny and Janie Churchill, 3136 Ellet Avenue, Akron, OH
44312. (216) 628-8335.
Support group for parents who have lost pregnancies or who have lost children during the
neonatal period.

CARE (Caring and Restoring Each Other)
c/o Irwin I. Weinfeld, M.D., Associate Director of Neonatal Intensive Care
Unit, The Toledo Hospital, 2142 North Cove Boulevard, Toledo, OH 43606.
(419) 473-4225.
Trained couples offer one-to-one support to parents, also monthly group meetings.

Compassionate Friends–Ohio
Chapters in Akron, Carrollton, Chagrin Falls/Cleveland, Cincinnati, Columbus, Dayton, Huber Heights/Dayton, Mt. Vernon, Niles, Parma/Cleve-
land, Westlake/Cleveland.
Contact National Headquarters for more information.

For Fathers of Children Who've Died
Contact Person: Rev. Ken Czillinger, St. Matthias Church, 1044 West Kempner Road, Cincinnati, OH 45240. (513) 851-1930.
Meets third Monday of every month at 8:00 P.M.

For Mothers of Children Who've Died
Contact Person: Claire Rebel, 3686 Donata Drive, Cincinnati, OH 45239. (513) 385-0592.
Meets first Tuesday of every month at 12:30 P.M.
Contact Person: Ruth Donnelly, 685 Lullaby Court, Cincinnati, OH 45238. (513) 451-3022.
Meets second Thursday of every month at 10:00 A.M.
Contact Person: Connie Baron, 793 Carini Lane, Cincinnati, OH 45218. (513) 825-3089.
Meets fourth Wednesday of every month at 10:00 A.M.

For Mothers of Children Who've Died During the First Year of Life
Contact Persons: Mary Jane Inglish, 2850 Resor Road, Fairfield, OH 45014. (513) 874-3315. Judy Sandquist, 6123 Fairway Drive, Cincinnati, OH 45212. (513) 631-7590.
Meets second Monday of every month at 8:00 P.M.

Mothers Supporting Mothers
Contact Persons: Carole Bonno, 902 Seton Avenue, Cincinnati, OH 45205. (513) 921-7690. Pat Stetter, 5890 Fourson Drive, Cincinnati, OH 45238. (513) 922-7896.
For women who have miscarried or experienced the death of a newborn.

PEND (Parents Experiencing Neonatal Death)
Rainbow Babies' and Children's Hospital, 2101 Adelbert Road, Cleveland, OH 44106. (216) 444-3753. Contact Person: Nancy Bartell.
Monthly meetings of parents' emotional support group.

Resolve, Inc.–Ohio
Chapters in Greater Cincinnati, Columbus.
Contact National Headquarters for more information.

SHARE
Marilyn Miller Graef, 1272 Indian Hill Drive, Bolivar, OH 44612. (216) 874-3100.

Support Groups for the Bereaved
Rev. Ken Czillinger, St. Matthias Church, 1044 West Kemper Road, Cincinnati, OH 45240. (513) 851-1930.
Father Czillinger has about a dozen groups. Contact him for details.

OKLAHOMA

AMEND
Cindy Wilcox, 1344 East 26th Place, Tulsa, OK 74100.

Compassionate Friends–Oklahoma
Chapters in Oklahoma City, Stillwater, Tulsa.
Contact National Headquarters for more information.

OREGON

Compassionate Friends–Oregon
Chapters in Albany, Eugene, Portland, Roseburg, Salem.
Contact National Headquarters for more information.

Resolve, Inc.–Oregon
Chapter in Portland.
Contact National Headquarters for more information.

PENNSYLVANIA

Compassionate Friends–Pennsylvania
Chapters in Ambler, Bala Cynwyd/Philadelphia, Beaver, Carlisle, Conneaut-
ville, Ebensburg, Ephrata, Harrisburg, Johnstown, Myerstown, Pittsburgh,
Warrington, West Chester, Wilkes-Barre, York.
Contact National Headquarters for more information.

Mary Ann Egges
10 Highland Court, Downington, PA 19335. (215) 269-9606.
Services to bereaved parents of newborns.

Grieving Process Group, Booth Maternity Center
Contact Person: Mr. Glen Lucas, 6051 Overbrook Avenue, Philadelphia, PA
19131. (215) 878-7800.
Individual, couple, or group counseling.

Chaplain Allen Helwig
Lebanon Valley General Hospital, 4th and Willow Streets, Lebanon, PA
17042. (717) 273-8521 (work). (717) 273-8926 (home).
Services to bereaved parents of newborns.

Pregnancy Loss Group
Medical Social Work Department, Magee Women's Hospital, Forbes Avenue
and Halket Street, Pittsburgh, PA 15213. (412) 647-4255.
Provides counseling services for individuals, couples and an ongoing group.

Resolve, Inc.–Pennsylvania
Chapters in Philadelphia, Pittsburgh.
Contact National Headquarters for more information.

SHARE
Donna and Joseph DeLuca, 60 Wren Way, Washington, PA 15301. (412) 745-7478. Kathy Kuhn, 418 Chelsea Drive, Lancaster, PA 17601. (717) 569-6059.

UNITE (Understanding Newborns in Traumatic Experiences)
Contact Person: Bernadette Foley, Director of Social Service, Jeanes Hospital, 7600 Central Avenue, Philadelphia, PA 19111. (215) 728-2082.
Support group for parents who have had miscarriage, stillbirth, or infant death up to 12 months. Provides group meetings and individual support. Twofold purpose: to educate the community and to provide parents with support.

RHODE ISLAND

Compassionate Friends–Rhode Island
Chapter in Pawtucket.
Contact National Headquarters for more information.

SOUTH CAROLINA

Compassionate Friends–South Carolina
Chapters in Charleston, Columbia.
Contact National Headquarters for more information.

SHARE
Deborah Finley, 1110 Hagood Avenue, Columbia, SC 29205. (803) 254-7132.

SOUTH DAKOTA

Resolve, Inc.–South Dakota
Chapter in Sioux Falls.
Contact National Headquarters for more information.

TENNESSEE

Compassionate Friends–Tennessee
Chapters in Clarksville, Memphis.
Contact National Headquarters for more information.

PEPD (Parents Experiencing Perinatal Death)
P. O. Box 38445, Germantown, TN 38138. (901) 767-8727.
Volunteer group of parents who provide emotional support to other parents whose babies have died as a result of premature death, stillbirth, or newborn death. Provides hospital visitation, telephone listening 24 hours a day, discussion groups, literature, and education.

Resolve, Inc.–Tennessee
Chapter in Nashville.
Contact National Headquarters for more information.

TEXAS

Bereaved Parent Support Group
Chaplain Raymond Wolfe, Methodist Hospital, P.O. Box 1201, 3615 19th
Street, Lubbock, TX 79408. (806) 792-1011.

Compassionate Friends–Texas
Chapters in Abilene, Austin, Dallas, Forth Worth, Houston, San Antonio.
Contact National Headquarters for more information.

Dennis and Lydia Schuetz
2105 Laurel, Bay City, TX 77414. (713) 245-7240.
Services to bereaved parents of newborns.

Forth Worth Children's Hospital
Contact Person: Sharon Whitney, A.C.S.W., 1400 Cooper, Forth Worth, TX
76104. (817) 336-9861.
Support services to bereaved parents of newborns.

HAND (HOPE's Aid in Neonatal Death)
Houston Organization for Parent Education, Inc., 3311 Richmond, Suite 330,
Houston, TX 77098. (713) 524-3089. Contact Person: Mrs. Karen P. Riley,
14207 Locke Lane, Houston, TX 77077. (713) 493-6792.
Support group for parents whose babies have died from the time of conception through
late infancy.

Resolve, Inc.–Texas
Chapter in San Antonio.
Contact National Headquarters for more information.

SHARE of San Antonio
Constance Clear, 3534 Avenue B, San Antonio, TX 78209. (512) 822-4135.

Sudden Infant Death
Harris County Health Department, P.O. Box 25249, Houston, TX 77005.

UTAH

Compassionate Friends–Utah
Chapter in Salt Lake City.
Contact National Headquarters for more information.

Resolve, Inc.–Utah
Chapter in Salt Lake City.
Contact National Headquarters for more information.

Sharing Heart
c/o Thomas D. Coleman, University of Utah Medical Center, Department of
Neonatology, Room 2B, 245, 50 North Medical Drive, Salt Lake City, UT
84132. (801) 581-7052.
*Support services for parents who have lost a pregnancy, a premature baby, or a newborn.
Both individual and group support available.*

VERMONT

Compassionate Friends–Vermont
Chapters in Newport, White River Junction.
Contact National Headquarters for more information.

Resolve, Inc.–Vermont
Chapter in Shelburne.
Contact National Headquarters for more information.

VIRGINIA

Compassionate Friends–Virginia
Chapters in Quantico, Tazewell.
Contact National Headquarters for more information.

WASHINGTON

Compassionate Friends–Washington
Chapters in Bothell/Seattle, Bremerton, Pullman, Spokane.
Contact National Headquarters for more information.

Parents of Prematures (Seattle)
Lauri Lowen, Chairman.
13613 N.E. 26th Place, Bellevue, WA 98005. (206) 883-6040. Branches in.
Port Angeles, Port Orchard.
*Parent support group, offering emotional and educational support to new parents ex-
periencing a high-risk birth.*

Parents of Stillborns
6210 S. 120th, Seattle, WA 98178. 3509 N.E. 33 Street, Tacoma, WA 98422.
(206) 772-5338. (206) 838-9833.
*Group of parents who have experienced the birth of a stillborn baby or neonatal death.
Offers hospital visits, telephone contact, monthly meetings, consultations, and referrals to
professional resources.*

WISCONSIN

AIID (Aid In Infant Death)

c/o Childbirth Education Association, Lynn Stathus, Educational Coordinator, 5636 W. Burleigh Street, Milwaukee, WI 53210. (414) 445-7470.

Support to parents who have experienced the death of an infant through miscarriage, prematurity, stillbirth, congenital defects, or any other cause.

Bereaved Parents Support Group,
Service of Childbirth Education Association of Madison

c/o Carol Fowler, 1016 Van Buren, Madison, WI 53711. (608) 257-6352.

Parent support groups: meetings twice a month, couples' group, women's group, bereaved parent packet (packet available, send $1.50). Telephone and letter friends, hospital visitors, and a lending library.

Compassionate Friends–Wisconsin

Chapters in Appleton, Green Bay, Milwaukee, Oshkosh, Ripon, Shawano, Waukesha, Whitefish Bay/Milwaukee.

Contact National Headquarters for more information.

Parents Supporting Parents

c/o Mary Berg, Rice Clinic, 2501 Main Street, Stevens Point, WI 54481. (715) 344-4120 or 4400.

Support service for parents; provides one-on-one support as well as groups.

Resolve, Inc.–Wisconsin

Chapter in Milwaukee.

Contact National Headquarters for more information.

Resolve Through Sharing

LaCrosse Lutheran Hospital, 1910 South Avenue, LaCrosse, WI 54601. (608) 785-0530, ext. 3454.

The Resolve Through Sharing program provides counseling and support, utilizing the one-to-one relationship of a trained counselor with specific knowledge of miscarriage, stillbirth, and neonatal death, as well as a parent support group.

SHARE

c/o Mari VandenBerg, Social Service Department, St. Vincent's Hospital, P.O. Box 1220, Green Bay, WI 54305. (414) 433-8261. St. Francis Medical Center, 700 West Avenue South, LaCrosse, WI 54601. (608) 785-0940. c/o Mary Koczan, St. Nicholas Hospital, 2419 Seamann Avenue, Sheboygan, WI 53081. (414) 459-8300.

Organizations Outside the United States

CANADA

Bereaved Families of Ontario
Diane Foster, Director, 214 Merton St., Suite 305, Toronto, Ontario M4S1A6.
(416) 481-3389.
Association of families who have lost a child through death.

Bereaved Parents of Windsor Infant Group
Canadian Mental Health Association
Contact Person: Kathy MacKendrick, 1226 Ouellette Avenue, Windsor, Ontario N8X1J5. (519) 254-2556.
A self-help organization offering individual and group services to those who have experienced a miscarriage, stillbirth, or perinatal death.

Canadian Foundation for the Study of Infant Death
181 Belsize Drive, Toronto, Ontario M4S-1L9. (416) 488-3260.
Offers support and information to families who have experienced SIDS, encourages public education, and supports education and research.

London Parents' Perinatal Association
Contact Person: Christine Isard, President, 70 Fiddlers Green, Unit 26, London, Ontario N6G 3G3. (519) 472-7457. Neonatal Intensive Care Unit, St. Joseph's Hospital, 268 Grosvenor Street, London, Ontario NGA 4V2 (519) 439-3271. Neonatal Intensive Care Unit, Victoria Hospital, 375 South Street, London, Ontario N6A 4G5. (519) 432-5241.
The association voluntarily supports the physicians and nurses working in the field of perinatal care with the objective of improving care of the high-risk pregnant woman and newborns who require the services of the intensive care nursery. Its objectives are parent support, educational seminars, fund-raising, and improving public awareness.

The Compassionate Friends–Winnipeg, Manitoba
National Center: 521 Montrose Street, Winnipeg, Manitoba R3M 3M3.

Parents Experiencing Perinatal Death Association (PEPDA)
c/o Gael Gilbert, 47 Alberta Avenue, Toronto, Ontario M6H 2R5. (416) 651-7422. c/o Judy Siegel, 136 Sunnyside Place, Dollard des Ormeaux, Quebec H9A 1V9.
Volunteer group of parents whose goal is to provide understanding and emotional support for other parents whose babies have died, whether as a result of prematurity, stillbirth, or newborn death.

Parents Support Group, St. Joseph's Hospital
Contact Persons: Mrs. Ardelle and Mr. Bill Sabo, 811 Westbury Crescent, London, Ontario N6J 3C8. (519) 618-3624.
Parents who have experienced a stillbirth, or the death of a newborn, volunteer to help other parents with the grief and with decisions associated with the death. Booklet, The Loss of Your Baby, *by Ardelle and Bill Sabo, available on request.*

Perinatal Support Group St. Joseph's Hospital
Contact Person: Director of Nurseries, Clinical Instructor Obstetrics, St. Joseph's Hospital, 268 Grosvenor Street, London, Ontario N6A 4V2. (519) 439-3271.
Physicians and nurses available on request to other physicians and nurses who wish support in caring for couples experiencing perinatal loss.

ENGLAND–UNITED KINGDOM

The Compassionate Friends–England
Contact Person: Charmion Mann, 25 Kingsdown Parade, Bristol BS6 5UE, 0272 74316

Foundation for the Study of Infant Death
c/o Lady Sylvia Limerick, 5th Floor, 4 Grosvenor Place, London SW1 7HD. (01) 235-1721.

MIND National Association for Mental Health
22 Harley Street, London W1N 1AE.

The National Stillbirth Study Group
24 Wimpole Street, London W1M 7AD.

The Stillbirth and Perinatal Death Association
15A. Christchurch Hill, London NW3 1JY. (01) 794-4601.

AUSTRALIA

AMEND
Mrs. Alice Coleman, 11 Parkland Drive, Wodonga, Victora 3690. 060 243679.
Provides telephone counseling and counseling for parents in the hospital. Education of professionals.

The Compassionate Friends
Lindsay and Margaret Harmer, 10 The Outlook, Glen Waverley, 3150, Victoria. (03) 232-8151.

NALAG (National Association of Loss and Grief)
Contact Person: Penny Cole, P.O. Box 129, Ashburton, 3147. 29 1651.
Branches in Victoria, New South Wales, Queensland, South Australia.
NALAG is a nonprofit organization that aims to promote better care and understanding of loss, grief, separation, and life-threatening illness as this is experienced by individuals, families, and service providers. Provides information resource and support groups for those who work with the dying and the bereaved and educational programs for professionals and the general public.

SANDS (Stillbirth and Neonatal Death Support)
Pam Roberts, Secretary, 280 French Street, Tuart Hill 6060, Western Australia. (09) 34975 21.
Group run by committee of six mothers. Provides education to professionals, phone contacts, monthly meeting and community educational meetings.
Contact Person: Mrs. Bronwyn Boulton, 26 Maldon Street, South Australia.

NEW ZEALAND

Bereaved Parents Group
2/5 Badderley Avenue, Kohimarama, Auckland 5.

Intercountry Adoption Resources

NEWSLETTERS, BOOKS, AND OTHER PUBLICATIONS

Amigos Newsletter. A Latin American adoptive parents' support group newsletter. 769 S.E. 37th, Hillsboro, OR 97123.

Gamines: How to Adopt from Latin America, by Jean Nelson-Erichsen and Heino R. Erichsen. Minneapolis: Dillon Press, 1980. Procedures for Latin American adoptions, information on 24 countries and 80 child-placing sources, bibliography. $13.95.

Handbook for Single Adoptive Parents. Committee for Single Adoptive Parents, P.O. Box 4074, Washington, DC 20015, 1980. $6.00.

How to Adopt from Asia, Europe, and the South Pacific, by Jean Nelson-Erichsen and Heino R. Erichsen, 1980. Order from Los Niños Publication, 919 W. 28th Street, Minneapolis, MN 55408. Covers 24 countries. Lists over 80 names and addresses of child-placing sources, plus procedures. $13.00.

National Directory of Intercountry Adoption Services Resources. U.S. Department of Health, Education and Welfare, Office of Human Development, DHEW Publ. No. (OHDS) 80-30252 (available from U.S. Government Printing Office, Washington, DC 20402). Lists agencies and parents' groups in all 50 states, Washington, D.C., and Puerto Rico.

News of OURS. OURS, Inc. (nationwide adoptive parents' group), 4711 30th Avenue South, Minneapolis, MN 55406. Excellent comprehensive source of information on ICA and articles about parents' experiences. $13.00 per year for membership and bimonthly newsletter/magazine.

Los Niños News. Edited by Jean Nelsen-Erichsen and Heino R. Erichsen. Bimonthly. $15.00 per year.

La Palabra. Published by Latin American Adoptive Parent Association, P.O. Box 72, Seaford, NY 11783. $5.00 for 6 issues.

Report on Foreign Adoptions. International Concerns Committee for Children (ICCC), 911 Cypress Drive, Boulder, CO 80303. Listing of approximately 60 contacts, agencies, and knowledgeable parent groups, with information on 30 countries. Reading list and basic ICA information. $8.00 per year with 9 monthly updates.

UNITED STATES–BASED INTERCOUNTRY ADOPTION AGENCIES

Crossroads, Inc.
4901 West 77th Street
Minneapolis, MN 55435
   Children from India, Colombia, Ecuador, El Salvador (latter three countries for Minnesota residents only)

Dillon Family and Youth Services, Inc.
2525 East 21st Street
Tulsa, OK 74114
   Korean children only

Friends of Children of Various Nations (FCVN)
600 Gilpin
Denver, CO 80218
   Children from Colombia, India, and Korea

Holt Adoption Program, Inc.
P.O. Box 2440
Eugene, OR 97402
   Children from India, Korea, Nicaragua, Philippines, Thailand

New Opportunities, Inc.
Box 1180
Orem, UT 84057
   Children from Chile

ADOPTIVE PARENTS' SUPPORT GROUPS

North American Council on Adoptable Children (NACAC)
1346 Connecticut Avenue, N.W. Suite 229
Washington, DC 20036
Newsletter $10.00 per year for 10 issues
  *Umbrella organization for linking adoptive parents' groups in the U.S. and Canada.
  Involved in children and family advocacy as well as public information and education.
  Maintains excellent current book list in the field of adoption.* To place book order:
  NACAC, 3900 Market St., Suite 247, Riverside, CA 92501.

Open Door Society
130 Temple Street
West Newton, MA 02165
(617) 969-7025
  Runs an adoption information service. Puts out a newsletter.

OURS, Inc.
4711 30th Avenue South
Minneapolis, MN 55406
  Nationwide adoptive parents' group. See publications.

Bibliography

THE EMOTIONAL AND PHYSICAL IMPACT OF LOSING A PREGNANCY

Becker, Ernest, *The Denial of Death.* New York: The Free Press, 1975.

Benedek, Therese, "The Psychobiology of Pregnancy," in *Parenthood: Its Psychology and Psychopathology,* ed. James Anthony and Theresa Benedek. Boston: Little, Brown, 1970.

Bibring, Grete L., *Some Considerations of the Psychological Processes in Pregnancy. Psychoanalytic Study of the Child,* vol. 14. New York: International University Press, 1959.

————, T. F. Dwyer, D. S. Huntington, and A. F. Valenstein, "A Study of the Psychological Processes in Pregnancy and of the Earliest Mother-Child Relationship. I. Some Propositions and Comments," in *Psychoanalytic Study of the Child,* vol. 16. New York: International Universities Press, 1961.

Boston Women's Health Collective, *Our Bodies, Ourselves.* New York: Simon and Schuster, 1976.

Bowlby, John, *Attachment and Loss.* New York: Basic Books, 1969.

————, "Process of Mourning," *Int. J. Psychoanal.* 42 (1961):317–340.

Brown, Norman O., *Life against Death.* New York: Vintage Books, 1959.

Cain, A. C., M. E. Erikson, I. Fast, and R. A. Vaughn, "Children's Disturbed Reactions to Their Mother's Miscarriage," *Psychosomatic Medicine* 24 (1964):58–66.

Chodorow, Nancy, *The Reproduction of Mothering.* Berkeley: University of California Press, 1978.

Corney, R. T., and F. T. Horton, Jr., "Pathological Grief Following Spontaneous Abortion," *Am. J. Psychiat.* 131 (1974):825–827.

Deutsch, Helene, *Motherhood.* Vol. 2 of Deutsch, *The Psychology of Women.* New York: Grune and Stratton, 1945.

Engel, George L., "Grief and Grieving," *Am. J. of Nursing,* 64 (1964):93–98

Feinbloom, Richard I., *Pregnancy, Birth, and the Newborn Baby.* New York: Dell, 1972.

Friedman, Rochelle R., and Karen A. Cohen, "Emotional Reactions to the Miscarriage of a Consciously Desired Pregnancy," in *The Woman Patient,* ed. Malkah Notman and Carol Nadelson, vol. 3. New York: Plenum Press, 1982.

————, "The Peer Support Group: A Model for Dealing with the Emotional Aspects of Miscarriage," *Group* 4 (1980):42–48.

Gaylin, Willard, *Caring*. New York: Avon, 1976.

Gradstein, Bonnie D., and Rhoda Levitt, *Guidelines for Pregnancy Counseling*. San Francisco: San Francisco Interagency Pregnancy Council, 1975. Distributed by Department of Health, Office of Planning.

Grimm, E. R., "Psychological Investigation of Habitual Abortion," *Psychosomatic Medicine* 24 (1962):369.

————, "Psychological Tension in Pregnancy," *Psychosomatic Medicine* 23 (1961):520–527.

Grossman, Frances Kaplan, Lois S. Eichler, Susan A. Winickoff, et al., *Pregnancy, Birth, and Parenthood*. San Francisco: Jossey-Bass, 1980.

Hamburg, D. A., and J. E. Adams, "A Perspective on Coping Behavior: Seeking and Utilizing Information in Major Transitions," *Arch. Gen. Psychiat.* 17 (1967):277–284.

Jessner, L., E. Weigert, and J. L. Foy, "The Development of Parental Attitudes during Pregnancy," in *Parenthood: Its Psychology and Psychopathology*, ed. James Anthony and Therese Benedek. Boston: Little, Brown, 1970.

Jessner, Lucie, "On Becoming a Mother," in *Conditio Humana*, ed. Walter von Baeyer and Richard M. Griffith. New York: Springer-Verlag, 1966.

Josselyn, Irene M., "Cultural Forces, Motherliness and Fatherliness," *Am. J. Orthopsychiatry* 26 (1945):264–271.

Kaij, L., A. Malmquist, and A. Nilsson, "Psychiatric Aspects of Spontaneous Abortion." II. The Importance of Bereavement, Attachment and Neurosis in Early Life," *J. of Psychosomatic Res.* 13 (1969):53–59.

Kennell, John H., Howard Slyter, and Marshall H. Klaus, "Mourning Response of Parents to the Death of a Newborn Infant," *NEJM* 283 (1970): 344–349.

Kestenberg, Judith S., "Regression and Reintegration in Pregnancy," *J. Am. Psychoanal. Assn.* 24 (1976): supplement, *Female Psychology*.

Klaus, Marshall H., and John H. Kennell, *Maternal-Infant Bonding*. St. Louis: Mosby, 1976.

Lennane, K. Jean and R. John, "Alleged Psychogenic Disorders in Women: A Possible Manifestation of Sexual Prejudice," *NEJM* 288 (1973).

Lindemann, Erich, "Symptomatology and Management of Acute Grief," *Am. J. of Psychiatry* 101 (1944):141.

McBride, A. B., *The Growth and Development of Mothers*. New York: Harper and Row, 1974.

McDonald, Ronald L., "The Role of Emotional Factors in Obstetric Complications: A Review," *Psychosomatic Medicine* 30 (1968):222–237.

Malmquist, A., L. Kaij, and A. Nilsson, "Psychiatric Aspects of Spontaneous Abortion. I. A Matched Control Study of Women with Living Children," *J. of Psychosomatic Res.* 13 (1969):45–51.

Menning, Barbara Eck, *Infertility: A Guide for the Childless Couple*. Englewood Cliffs: Prentice-Hall, 1977.

Michel-Wolfromm, H., "The Psychological Factor in Spontaneous Abortion," *J. of Psychosomatic Res.* 12 (1968):67–71.

Miller, Rita S., "The Social Construction and Reconstruction of Physiologic Events: Acquiring the Pregnancy Identity" in Norman K. Denzin (ed.), *Studies in Symbolic Interaction*, vol. 1. (1978), pp. 181–204.

Parkes, C. Murray, "The Nature of Grief," *Int. J. of Psychiatry* 3 (1967):435–438.

Pohlman, Edward, *The Psychology of Birth Planning*. Cambridge, Mass.: Schenkman, 1969.

Pollock, G., "Mourning and Adaptation," *Int. J. Psychoanal.* 42 (1961):341–361.

Russell, Keith P., *Eastman's Expectant Motherhood*, 7th ed. Boston: Little, Brown, 1980.

Sander, W., "Adaptive Relationships in Early Mother-Child Interaction," *J. Am. Acad. Child Psychiatry*, 3 (1964):231–265.

Seibel, Machelle, and William L. Graves, "The Psychological Implications of Spontaneous Abortion," *J. of Reprod. Medicine* 25 (1980):161–165.

Sherman, Julia A., "Pregnancy," *On the Psychology of Woman: A Survey of Empirical Studies*. Illinois: Charles C. Thomas, 1973.

Siggins, Lorraine D., "Mourning: A Critical Survey of the Literature," *Int. J. Psychoanal.* 47 (1966):14–25.

Simon, N. M., P. Rothman, J. T. Goff, et al., "Psychological Factors Related to Spontaneous and Therapeutic Abortion," *Am. J. Obs. and Gyn.* 104 (1969): 799–806.

Solnit, Albert J., and Mary H. Stark, *Mourning and the Birth of a Defective Child, Psychoanalytic Study of the Child*, vol. 16. New York: International University Press (1961).

Stack, Jack M., "Spontaneous Abortion and Grieving," *American Family Physician* 21 (1980):99–102.

Tupper, C., et al., "The Problem of Spontaneous Abortion," *Am. J. Obs. and Gyn.* 73 (1957):313.

Winnicott, D. W., "The Theory of Parent-Infant Relationship," in *The Maturational Process and the Facilitating Environment*, ed. D. W. Winnicott. New York: International Universities Press, 1965.

Yalom, Irvin D., et al., "Postpartum Blues Syndrome," *Arch. Gen. Psychiatry* 18 (1968):16–27.

MISCARRIAGE

Alberman, E., et al., "Previous Reproductive History in Mothers Presenting with Spontaneous Abortions," *Brit. J. Obs. and Gyn.* 82 (1975):366.

Assali, Nicholas S., ed., *Pathophysiology of Gestation*, vol. 2. New York: Academic Press, 1972.

Barnes, Ann B., et al., "Fertility and Outcome of Pregnancy in Women Exposed in Utero to Diethylstilbestrol," *NEJM* 302, No. 11 (1980):609–613.

Bennett, M. J., and R. H. J. Kerr-Wilson, "Evaluation of Threatened Abortion by Ultrasound," *Int. J. Gyn. and Obs.* 17 (1980):382–384.

Byrd, J. Rogers, et al., "Cytogenic Findings in Fifty-five Couples with Recurrent Fetal Wastage," *Fertility and Sterility* 28 (1977):246–250.

Cain, Albert C., et al., "Children's Disturbed Reactions to Their Mother's Miscarriage," *Psychosomatic Medicine* 26 (1964):58–66.

Carr, D. H., "Chromosome Anomalies as a Cause of Spontaneous Abortion," *Am. J. Obs. and Gyn.* 97 (1967):283–293.

———, "Genetic Basis of Abortion," *Annual Rev. of Genetics* 5 (1971):64.

Clapp, Diane, "Luteal Phase Defect," *RESOLVE Newsletter*, September 1980.

———, "T-Mycoplasm: Its Role in Infertility and Miscarriage," *RESOLVE Newsletter*, June, 1979.

Danforth, David N., ed., *Obstetrics and Gynecology*, 3rd ed. New York: Harper and Row, 1977.

Fabricant, Jill D., et al., "Cytogenetic Abnormalities in Spontaneous Abortion" in *Management of High Risk Pregnancy*, ed. John T. Queenan. Oradell: Medical Economics, 1980.

――――, "Genetic Studies on Spontaneous Abortion," *Contemporary Obs. and Gyn.* 11 (1978):73–78.

Glass, Robert H., ed.., *Office Gynecology*, 2nd ed. Baltimore: Williams and Wilkins, 1981.

―――― and Mitchell S. Golbus, "Habitual Abortion," *Fertility and Sterility* 29 (1978):257–265.

Gnarpe, H., and J. Friberg, "Mycoplasma and Human Reproduction Failure," *Am. J. Obs. and Gyn.* 114 (1972):727.

Goldstein, Donald P., and Merle J. Berger, "Reproductive Failure in DES-Exposed Women," *RESOLVE Newsletter*, June 1980.

Grimm, Elaine R., "Psychological Investigation of Habitual Abortion," *Psychosomatic Medicine* 24 (1962):369–378.

――――, and Wanda R. Venet, "The Relationship of Emotional Adjustment and Attitudes to the Course and Outcome of Pregnancy," *Psychosomatic Medicine* 28 (1966):34–49.

Guerrero, R., and O. I. Rojas, "Spontaneous Abortion and Aging of Human Ova and Spermatozoa," *NEJM* 293 (1975):573.

Hertiz, A. T., and R. G. Livingstone, "Spontaneous Threatened and Habitual Abortion: Their Prognosis and Treatment," *NEJM* 230 (1944):798.

James, William H., "The Problem of Spontaneous Abortion," *Am J. Obs. and Gyn.* 85 (1963):38–40.

Kajii, Tadashi, and Ariane Ferrier, "Cytogenetics of Aborters and Abortuses," *Am. J. Obs. and Gyn.* 131 (1978):33.

Kline, J., "Smoking a Risk Factor for Spontaneous Abortion," *NEJM* 297 (1977):793–796.

Malmquist, A., L. Kaij, and A. Nilsson, "Psychiatric Aspects of Spontaneous Abortion. I. A Matched Control Study of Women with Living Children," *J. of Psychosomatic Res.* 13 (1969):45–51.

Menning, Barbara Eck, and Diane Clapp, "The Emotional Impact of Miscarriage," *RESOLVE Newsletter*, September 1979.

Michel-Wolfromm, H., "The Psychological Factor in Habitual Abortion," *J. of Psychosomatic Res.* 12 (1968):67–71.

Newton, Niles, "Emotions of Pregnancy," *Clinical Obs. and Gyn.* 6 (1963):638–668.

Niswander, Kenneth R., *Obstetrics: Essentials of Clinical Practice*, 2nd ed. Boston: Little, Brown, 1981.

Patterson, Sam P., and William T. Black, Jr., "When Women Habitually Abort," *Postgraduate Medicine* 43(1968):59–66.

Schweditsch, M. O., "Hormonal Considerations in Early Normal Pregnancy and Blighted Ovum Syndrome," *Fertility and Sterility* 31 (1979):252–257.

Seibel, Machelle, and William L. Graves, "The Psychological Implications of Spontaneous Abortion," *J. of Reproductive Medicine* 25 (1980):161–165.

Sher, G., "Induction of Labor Following Intrauterine Death with Intra-amniotic Hyperosmolar Urea and Prostaglandin F_2: Evaluation of Placental Endocrine Function and Changes in Coagulation Parameters," *Am. J. Obs. and Gyn.* 134 (1979):493–497.

Simon, N. M., et al., "Psychological Factors Related to Spontaneous and Therapeutic Abortion," *Am. J. Obs. and Gyn.* 104 (1969):799–806.
Speroff, L., R. H. Glass, and N. Kase, *Clinical Gynecologic Endocrinology and Infertility,* 2nd ed. Baltimore: Williams and Wilkins, 1978.
Stack, Jack, "Spontaneous Abortion and Grieving," *Am. Fa· 1   Physician* 21 (1980):99–102.
Surgeon General's Advisory on Alcohol and Pregnancy. *FDA Drug Bulletin* 11 (July 1981).
Taylor, E. Stewart, ed., *Beck's Obstetrical Practice and Fetal Medicine.* Baltimore: Williams and Wilkins, 1976.
Tho, Phung T., J. R. Byrd, and P. G. McDonough, "Etiologies and Subsequent Reproductive Performance of 100 Couples with Recurrent Abortion," *Fertility and Sterility* 32 (1979):389–395
Tupper, C., et al., "The Problem of Spontaneous Abortion," *Am. J. Obs. and Gyn.* 73 (1957):313–321
Weathersbee, P. S., et al., "Caffeine in Pregnancy," *Postgraduate Medicine* 62 (1977):64–69

STILLBIRTH

Anonymous, "The Abhorrence of Stillbirth," *The Lancet* (1977):1188–1190.
———, "Easing the Pain and Grief of Stillbirth," *Nursing Mirror* 146 (June 1, 1978):38–41.
Beard, R. W., et al., "Help for Parents after Stillbirth," *Brit. Medical J.* 1 (1978):172–173.
Beischer, N. A., and E. V. Mackay, "Ultrasonic Echography," in *Obstetrics and the Newborn.* Philadelphia: Saunders, 1976.
Bourne, Stanford, "The Psychological Effects of Stillbirths on the Doctor." *Proceedings,* Third International Congress of Psychosomatic Medicine in Obstetrics and Gynaecology, London, 1971, pp. 333–334.
———, "The Psychological Effects of Stillbirths on Women and Their Doctors," *J. Royal College of General Practitioners* 16 (1968):103–112.
Breuer, Judith, "Sharing a Tragedy," *Am. J. Nursing* 76 (1976):758–759.
Clarke, Michael, "Depression in Women after Perinatal Death," *The Lancet* 1 (1979):916–917.
Cullberg, J., "Mental Reactions of Women to Perinatal Death," *Proceedings,* Third International Congress of Psychosomatic Medicine in Obstetrics and Gynaecology, London, 1971, pp. 326–329.
Danforth, David N., ed., *Obstetrics and Gynecology,* 3rd ed. New York: Harper and Row, 1977.
Dunlop, Joyce, "Bereavement Reaction Following Stillbirth," *The Practitioner* 222 (1979):115–118.
Engel, George L., "Grief and Grieving," *Am. J. Nursing* 64 (1964):93–98.
Fedrick, Jean, and Philippa Adelstein, "Influences of Pregnancy Spacing on Outcome of Pregnancy," *Brit. J. Medicine* 29 (1973):753–756.
Giles, P. F. H., "Reactions of Women to Perinatal Death," *Australian and New Zealand J. of Obs. and Gyn.* 10 (1970):207–210.
Goplerud, Clifford P., "Bleeding in Late Pregnancy," in *Obstetrics and Gynecology,* 3rd ed., ed. David N. Danforth. New York: Harper and Row, 1977. Pp. 378–387.

Hallett, Elizabeth R., "Birth and Grief," *Birth and the Family J.* 1 (1974):18–22.

Hardgrove, Carol, and Louise Warrick, "How Shall We Tell the Children?" *Am. J. Nursing* 74 (1974):448–450.

Jolly, Hugh, "Family Reactions to Child Bereavement," *Proceedings* of the Royal Society of Medicine 69 (1976):835–842.

———, "Loss of a Baby," *Australian Pediatric J.* 14 (1978):3–5.

Kennell, John H., et al., "The Mourning Response of Parents to the Death of a Newborn Infant," *NEJM* 283 (1976):344–346.

Knapp, Ronald J., and Larry G. Peppers, "Doctor-Patient Relationships in Fetal/Infant Death Encounters," *J. Medical Education* 54 (1979):775–780.

Kotzwinkle, William, "Swimmer in the Secret Sea," *Redbook Magazine,* July 1974.

Laursen, N. H., et al., "Management of Intrauterine Fetal Death with Prostaglandins E_2 Vaginal Suppositories," *Am. J. Obs. and Gyn.* 137 (1980): 753–757.

Lewis, B. Victor, et al., "Vaginal Breech Delivery or Cesarean Section?" *Am. J. Obs. and Gyn.* 134 (1979):615–618.

Lewis, Emanuel, "The Management of Stillbirth: Coping with an Unreality," *The Lancet* 2 (1976):619–620.

———, "Mourning by the Family after a Stillbirth or Neonatal Death," *Archives of Disease in Childhood* 54 (1979):303–306.

———, "Reactions to Stillbirth," *Proceedings,* Third International Congress of Psychosomatic Medicine in Obstetrics and Gynaecology, London, 1971, pp. 323–325.

———, and Anne Page, "Failure to Mourn a Stillbirth: An Overlooked Catastrophe," *Brit. J. Medical Psychology* 51 (1978):237–241.

Lindemann, Erich, "Symptomatology and Management of Acute Grief," *Am. J. Psychiat.* 101 (1944):141–148.

Mann, Leon L., "Modern Management of the Breech Delivery," *Am. J. Obs. and Gyn.* 134 (1979): 611–614.

Newton, Michael, "Other Complications of Labor," in *Obstetrics and Gynecology,* 3rd ed., ed. David L. Danforth. New York: Harper and Row, 1977.

Parkes, C. Murray, "The Nature of Grief," *Int. J. Psychiat.* 3 (1967):435–438.

Poznanski, Elva Orlow, "The Replacement Child: A Saga of Unresolved Parental Grief," *J. Pediatrics* 81 (1972):1191–1193.

Ross, Tamara, "Stillbirth: A New Approach." Interview with Hugh Jolly, *Nursing Mirror* 143 (1976):40–41.

Rowe, J., et al., "Followup: Families Who Experience a Perinatal Death," *J. Pediatrics* 62 (1978):166–170.

Seitz, Pauline M., and Louise H. Warrick, "Perinatal Death: The Grieving Mother," *Am. J. Nursing* 74 (1974):2028–2033.

Sher, G., "Induction of Labor Following Intrauterine Death with Intraamniotic Hypersmolar Urea and Prostaglandin F_2 α: Evaluation of Placental Endocrine Function and Changes in Coagulation Parameters," *Am. J. Obs. and Gyn.* 134 (1979).

Sonstegard, Lois, et al., "The Grieving Nurse," *Am J. Nursing* 76 (1976):1490–1492.

Speck, William T., "Commentary: The Tragedy of Stillbirth," *J. Pediatrics* 93 (1978):869–870.

Taylor, E. Stewart, ed., *Beck's Obstetrical Practive and Fetal Medicine.* Baltimore: Williams and Wilkins, 1976.

Wolff, John R., "The Emotional Reaction to a Stillbirth." *Proceedings,* Third International Congress of Psychosomatic Medicine in Obstetrics and Gynaecology, London, 1971. Pp. 330–332.
———, et al., "The Emotional Reaction to a Stillbirth," *Am. J. Obs. and Gyn.* 108 (1970):73–77.
Worlow, Dorothy, "What Do You Say When the Baby Is Stillborn?" *RN* 41 (1978):74.

ECTOPIC PREGNANCY

Bender, S., "Fertility after Tubal Pregnancy," *Brit. J. Obs. and Gyn.* 63 (1956):400.
Boyd, J. E., and E. M. Holt, "Tubal Sterility, Patency Tests, and Results of Operation," *Brit. J. Obs. and Gyn.* 80 (1973):142.
Bukovsky, I., et al., "Conservative Surgery for Tubal Pregnancy," *Obs. and Gyn.* 53 (1979):709–711.
Franklin, E. W. III, A. M. Zeiderman, and P. Laemmle, "Tubal Ectopic Pregnancy: Etiology and Obstetric and Gynecologic Sequelae," *A. J. Obs. and Gyn.* 117 (1973):220.
Glass, Robert H., *Office Gynecology,* 2nd ed. Baltimore: Williams and Wilkins, 1981.
Hallatt, J. G., "Repeat Ectopic Pregnancy: A Study of 123 Consecutive Cases," *Am. J. Obs. and Gyn.* 122 (1975):520.
Kitchin, James D. III, et al., "Ectopic Pregnancy: Current Clinical Trends," *Am. J. Obs. and Gyn.* 134 (1979):870.
Schenker, J. G., et al., "Fertility after Tubal Pregnancy," *Surg. Gyn. and Obs.* 135 (1972):74–76.
Schoen, J. A., and R. J. Nowak, "Repeat Ectopic Pregnancy," *Obs. and Gyn.* 45 (1975):542–546.
Skulj, V., Z. Pavlic, C. Stoilkovic, et al., "Conservative Operative Treatment of Tubal Pregnancy," *Fertility and Sterility* 15 (1964):634.
Toaff, R., "Disturbances of Gestational Potency," in Charles A. Joel, *Fertility Disturbances in Men and Women.* New York: S. Karger, 1971.

MULTIPLE LOSSES

Berger, M., and D. Goldstein, "Impaired Reproductive Performance in DES-Exposed Women," *Obs. and Gyn.* 55 (1980):25–27.
Danforth, David N., ed., *Obstetrics and Gynecology,* 3rd ed. New York: Harper and Row, 1977.
Glass, R. H., and M. S. Golbus, "Habitual Abortion," *Fertility and Sterility* 29 (1978): 257–265.
Grimm, Elaine R., "Psychological Investigation of Habitual Abortion," *Psychosomatic Medicine* 24 (1962):369–378.
Hendin, David, and Joan Marks, *The Genetic Connection.* New York: Signet, 1979.
Hertz, Dan G., "Rejection of Motherhood," *Psychosomatics* 14 (1973):241–244.
Mazor, M., "The Problem of Infertility," in *The Woman Patient,* vol. 1, ed. Malkah Notman and Carol Nadelson. New York: Plenum Press, 1978.
——— "Barren Couples," *Psychology Today,* May 1979.

Menning, Barbara Eck, *Infertility: A Guide for the Childless Couple.* Englewood Cliffs: Prentice-Hall, 1978.
————, "Counseling Infertile Couples," *Contemporary Obs. and Gyn.* 13 (1979):101–108.
————, "The Emotional Needs of Infertile Couples," *Fertility and Sterility* 34 (1980):313–319.
Niswander, Kenneth R., *Obstetrics: Essentials of Clinical Practice,* 2nd ed. Boston: Little, Brown, 1981.
Patterson, Sam P., and William T. Black, Jr., "When Women Habitually Abort," *Postgraduate Medicine* 43 (1968):59–66.
Rosenfeld, D. L., and E. Mitchell, "Treating the Emotional Aspects of Infertility: Counseling Services in an Infertility Clinic," *Am. J. Obs. and Gyn.* 135 (1979):177–180.
Speroff, L., R. H. Glass, and N. G. Kase, *Clinical Gynecologic Endocrinology and Infertility,* 2nd ed. Baltimore: Williams and Wilkins, 1978.
Stangel, John J., *Fertility and Conception: An Essential Guide for Childless Couples.* New York: Paddington Press, 1979.
Taylor, E. Stewart, ed., *Beck's Obstetrical Practice and Fetal Medicine.* Baltimore: Williams and Wilkins, 1976.
Tho, Phung T., J. Rogers Byrd, and Paul G. McDonough, "Etiologies and Subsequent Reproductive Performance of 100 Couples with Recurrent Abortion," *Fertility and Sterility* 32 (1979):389–395.

THE HUSBAND'S EXPERIENCE

Freeman, T., "Pregnancy as a Precipitant of Mental Illness in Men," *Brit. J. Medical Psychol.* 24 (1951):49.
"Grieving after Spontaneous Abortion Often Unrecognized," *Obs. Gyn. News,* 14 (1981):31.
Group for the Advancement of Psychiatry, Committee in Public Education, *The Joys and Sorrows of Parenthood.* New York: Charles Scribner's Sons, 1973.
Jarvis, W., "Some Effects of Pregnancy and Childbirth on Men," *J. Am. Psychoanal. Assn.* 10 (1962):689–700.
Josselyn, Irene M., "Cultural Forces, Motherliness and Fatherliness," *Am. J. Orthopsychiatry* 26 (1956):264–271.
Kennell, John H., Howard Slyter, and Marshall H. Klaus, "The Mourning Response of Parents to the Death of a Newborn," *NEJM* 283 (1970): 344–349.
Pleck, Joseph H., and Jack Sawyer, eds., *Men and Masculinity.* Englewood Cliffs: Prentice-Hall, 1974.
Zilboorg, Gregory, "Depressive Reactions Related to Parenthood," *Am. J. Psychiat.* 10 (1931):927–962.

FAMILY AND FRIENDS: REACTIONS OF AND REACTIONS TO

Cain, Albert C., et al., "Children's Disturbed Reactions to Their Mothers' Miscarriage," *Psychosomatic Medicine* 24 (1964):58–66.
Cain, Albert C., I. Fast, and M. E. Erickson, "Children's Disturbed Reactions to the Death of a Sibling," *Am J. Orthopsychiatry* 34 (1964):741–752.

Cain, A. C., et al., "On Replacing a Child," *J. Am. Acad. Child Psychiatry* 3 (1964):443–456.

Hardgrove, Carol, and Louise H. Warrick, "How Shall We Tell the Children?" *Am. J. Nursing* 74 (1974):448–450.

Jolly, Hugh, "Family Reactions to Child Bereavement," *Proceedings* of the Royal Society of Medicine 69 (1976):835–842.

———, "Loss of a Baby," *Australian Pediatric J.* 14 (1978):3–5.

Klaus, Marshall H., and John H. Kennell, *Maternal-Infant Bonding*. St. Louis: Mosby, 1976.

Lewis, Emanuel, "Mourning by the Family after a Stillbirth or Neonatal Death," *Archives of Disease of Childhood* 54 (1979):303–306.

———, "Reactions to Stillbirth," *Proceedings,* International Congress of Psychosomatic Medicine in Obstetrics and Gynaecology, Third International Congress. Basel: Karger, 1972.

Nagera, Humberto, "Children's Reactions to the Death of Important Objects: A Development Approach," in *The Psychoanalytical Study of the Child,* vol. 25. New York: International Universities Press, 1970.

BOOKS ON DEATH FOR CHILDREN (AND PARENTS)

Primary Grades and Preschool

De Bruyn, M. G., *The Beaver Who Wouldn't Die.* Chicago: Follett, 1975.

Fassler, Joan, *My Grandpa Died Today.* New York: Behavioral Publications, 1971.

Viorst, Judith, *The Tenth Good Thing about Barney.* New York: Atheneum, 1971.

Children 10 to 14 Years Old

Miles, Betty, *The Trouble with Thirteen.* New York: Knopf, 1979.

Paterson, Katherine, *The Bridge to Terabithia.* New York: Crowell, 1977.

Parents and Children

Zim, Herbert S., and Sonia Bleeker, *Life and Death.* New York: Morrow, 1970.

Parents

Grollman, Earl, *Explaining Death to Children.* Boston: Beacon Press, 1969.

Rudolph, Marguerite, *Should the Children Know? Encounters with Death in the Lives of Children.* New York: Schocken, 1978.

Wolf, Anna W. M., ed., *Helping Your Child to Understand Death.* Child Study Association of America, 1958.

PLANNING FOR THE FUTURE

"AMA Labels Marijuana as Dangerous Drug," *Psychiatric News,* April 17, 1981.

Bernard, J., *The Future of Motherhood.* New York: Penguin, 1975.

Clarren, Sterling K., and David W. Smith, "The Fetal Alcohol Syndrome," *NEJM* 298 (1978):1063–1067.

Daniels, P., and K. Weingarten, "A New Look at the Medical Risks in Late
    Childbearing," *Women and Health* 4 (1979):5–35.
Dywasuk, Colette T., *Adoption: Is It for You?* New York: Harper and Row, 1973.
Fedrick, Jean, and Philippa Adelstein, "Influence of Pregnancy Spacing on
    Outcome of Pregnancy," *British Med. J.* 4 (1973):753–756.
Gradstein, B., M. Gradstein, and R. Glass, "Private Adoption," *Fertility and
    Sterility* 37 (1982).
Harrison, Mary, *Infertility: A Guide for Couples.* Boston: Houghton Mifflin, 1979.
Martin, Cynthia, *Beating the Adoption Game.* La Jolla: Oak Tree, 1980.
McNamara, Joan, *The Adoption Advisor.* New York: Hawthorne Books, 1975.
Menning, Barbara Eck, *Infertility: A Guide for Childless Couples.* Englewood
    Cliffs: Prentice-Hall, 1978.
Perkins, Richard P., "Sexual Behavior and Response in Relation to Compli-
    cations of Pregnancy," *Am. J. Obs. and Gyn.* 134 (1979):498–505.
Poznanski, Elva Orlow, "The Replacement Child: A Saga of Unresolved Pa-
    rental Grief," *J. Pediatrics* 81 (1972):1190–1193.
"Pregnancy: The Ultimate Goal," *RESOLVE Newsletter,* Sept. 1980.
Raymond, Louise, *Adoption and After.* New York: Harper and Row, 1974.
Sorosky, Arthur D., A. Baran, and R. Pannor, *The Adoption Triangle.* New
    York: Doubleday/Anchor, 1978.
Speroff, L., R. H. Glass, and N. G. Kase, *Clinical Gynecologic Endocrinology and
    Infertility.* 2nd ed. Baltimore: Williams and Wilkins, 1978.
Surgeon General's Advisory on Alcohol and Pregnancy, *FDA Drug Bulletin,* 11
    (1981):1.

Index